AGING ISSUES, HEALTH AND FINANCIAL ALTERNATIVES

NURSING HOMES: QUALITY AND CARE ISSUES

AGING ISSUES, HEALTH AND FINANCIAL ALTERNATIVES

Additional books in this series can be found on Nova's website under the Series tab.

Additional E-books in this series can be found on Nova's website under the E-books tab.

AGING ISSUES, HEALTH AND FINANCIAL ALTERNATIVES

NURSING HOMES: QUALITY AND CARE ISSUES

CARLOS E. MELENDEZ
EDITOR

Nova
Nova Science Publishers, Inc.
New York

For permission to use material from this book please contact us:
Telephone 631-231-7269; Fax 631-231-8175
Web Site: http://www.novapublishers.com

LIBRARY OF CONGRESS CATALOGING-IN-PUBLICATION DATA
Nursing homes : quality and care issues / editor, Carlos E. Melendez.
p. cm.
Includes index.
ISBN 978-1-61668-855-4 (hardcover)
1. Nursing homes--Quality control. I. Melendez, Carlos E.
RA997.N9 2009
362.16068--dc22
2010012884

Published by Nova Science Publishers, Inc. ✦ New York

CONTENTS

PREFACE

The nation's 1.5 million nursing home residents are a highly vulnerable population of elderly and disabled individuals for whom remaining at home is no longer feasible. With the aging of the baby boom generation, the number of individuals needing nursing home care and the associated costs are expected to increase dramatically. The federal government plays a key role in ensuring that nursing home residents receive appropriate care by setting quality-of-care, quality-of-life, and life safety requirements that nursing homes must meet to participate in the Medicare and Medicaid programs and by contracting with states to encourage compliance with these requirements, Congress has authorized certain enforcement actions. This book addresses and evaluates the quality of nursing home care across the nation and explores the enforcement and oversight functions intended to ensure high-quality care.

Chapter 1 - With the Omnibus Budget Reconciliation Act of 1987 (OBRA '87), Congress responded to growing concerns about the quality of care that nursing home residents received by requiring reforms in the federal certification and oversight of nursing homes. These reforms included revising care requirements that homes must meet to participate in the Medicare or Medicaid programs, modifying the survey process for certifying a home's compliance with federal standards, and introducing additional sanctions and decertification procedures for noncompliant homes.

GAO's testimony addresses its work in evaluating the quality of nursing home care and the enforcement and oversight functions intended to ensure high- quality care, the progress made in each of these areas since the passage of OBRA '87, and the challenges that remain.

GAO's testimony is based on its prior work; analysis of data from the Centers for Medicare & Medicaid Services' (CMS) On-Line Survey, Certification, and Reporting system (OSCAR), which compiles the results of state nursing home surveys; and evaluation of federal comparative surveys for selected states (2005- 2007). Federal comparative surveys are conducted at nursing homes recently surveyed by each state to assess the adequacy of the state's surveys.

Chapter 2 - Under contract with the CMS, states conduct surveys at nursing homes to help ensure compliance with federal quality standards. Over the past decade, GAO has reported on inconsistencies in states' assessment of nursing homes' quality of care, including understatement—that is, when state surveys fail to cite serious deficiencies or cite them at too low a level. In 2008, GAO reported that 9 states had high and 10 had low understatement based on CMS data for fiscal years 2002 through 2007. This chapter examines the effect on nursing home deficiency understatement of CMS's survey process, workforce shortages and training, supervisory reviews of surveys, and state agency practices. GAO primarily collected data through two Web-based questionnaires sent to all eligible nursing home surveyors and state agency directors, achieving 61 and 98 percent response rates, respectively.

Chapters 3 through 11 feature testimony before a government committee.

In: Nursing Homes Quality and Care Issues
Editor: Carlos E. Melendez
ISBN: 978-1-61668-855-4

Chapter 1

NURSING HOME REFORM: CONTINUED ATTENTION IS NEEDED TO IMPROVE QUALITY OF CARE IN A SMALL BUT SIGNIFICANT SHARE OF HOMES*

Kathryn G. Allen

WHY GAO DID THIS STUDY

With the Omnibus Budget Reconciliation Act of 1987 (OBRA '87), Congress responded to growing concerns about the quality of care that nursing home residents received by requiring reforms in the federal certification and oversight of nursing homes. These reforms included revising care requirements that homes must meet to participate in the Medicare or Medicaid programs, modifying the survey process for certifying a home's compliance with federal standards, and introducing additional sanctions and decertification procedures for noncompliant homes.

GAO's testimony addresses its work in evaluating the quality of nursing home care and the enforcement and oversight functions intended to ensure high- quality care, the progress made in each of these areas since the passage of OBRA '87, and the challenges that remain.

GAO's testimony is based on its prior work; analysis of data from the Centers for Medicare & Medicaid Services' (CMS) On-Line Survey, Certification, and Reporting system (OSCAR), which compiles the results of state nursing home surveys; and evaluation of federal comparative surveys for selected states (2005- 2007). Federal comparative surveys are conducted at nursing homes recently surveyed by each state to assess the adequacy of the state's surveys.

www.gao.gov/cgi-bin/getrpt?GAO-07-794T.

To view the full product, including the scope and methodology, click on the link above. For more information, contact Kathryn G. Allen at (202) 512-7118 or allenk@gao.gov.

---

* This is an edited, reformatted and augmented version of a U. S. Government Accountability Office publication dated May 2007.

WHAT GAO FOUND

The reforms of OBRA '87 and subsequent efforts by CMS and the nursing home industry to improve the quality of nursing home care have focused on resident outcomes, yet a small but significant share of nursing homes nationwide continue to experience quality-of-care problems. In fiscal year 2006, almost one in five nursing homes was cited for serious deficiencies, those that caused actual harm or placed residents in immediate jeopardy. While this rate has fluctuated over the last 7 years, GAO has found persistent variation in the proportion of homes with serious deficiencies across states. In addition, although the understatement of serious deficiencies—that is, when federal surveyors identified deficiencies that were missed by state surveyors—has declined since 2004 in states GAO reviewed, it has continued at varying levels.

CMS has strengthened its enforcement capabilities since OBRA '87 in order to better ensure that nursing homes achieve and maintain high-quality care, but several key initiatives require refinement. CMS has implemented additional sanctions authorized in the legislation, established an immediate sanctions policy for homes found to repeatedly harm residents, and developed a new enforcement management data system. However, the immediate sanctions policy is complex and appears to have induced only temporary compliance in some homes with a history of repeated noncompliance. Furthermore, CMS's new data system's components are not integrated and national reporting capabilities are incomplete, which hamper CMS's ability to track and monitor enforcement.

CMS oversight of nursing home quality has increased significantly, but CMS initiatives continue to compete for staff and financial resources. Attention to oversight has led to greater demand on limited resources, and to queues and delays in certain key initiatives. For example, a new survey methodology has been in development for over 8 years and resource constraints threaten the planned expansion of this methodology beyond the initial demonstration states.

Significant attention from the Special Committee on Aging, the Institute of Medicine, and others served as a catalyst to focus national attention on nursing home quality issues, culminating in the nursing home reform provisions of OBRA '87. In response to many GAO recommendations and at its own initiative, CMS has taken many important steps; however, the task of ensuring high-quality nursing home care for all residents is not complete. In order to guarantee that all nursing home residents receive high-quality care, it is important to maintain the momentum begun by the reforms of OBRA '87 and continue to focus national attention on those homes that cause actual harm to vulnerable residents.

Mr. Chairman and Members of the Committee:

I am pleased to be here today as you acknowledge the 20th anniversary of the passage of the Omnibus Budget Reconciliation Act of 1987 (OBRA '87), which contained nursing home reform provisions. In March 1986, the National Academy of Sciences' Institute of Medicine (IOM) released a report concluding that quality of care and quality of life in many nursing homes were not satisfactory, despite the existence of government regulation, and that more effective government regulation could substantially improve nursing home quality.[1] In July 1987, we issued a report recommending that Congress pass legislation that would strengthen enforcement of federal nursing home requirements, consistent with the IOM's recommendations.[2] Largely in response to these reports, Congress passed the nursing home reform provisions of OBRA '87, which was significant in that it changed the focus of quality standards from a home's capability to provide care to its actual delivery of care and resident outcomes. OBRA '87 directed the Health Care Financing Administration, now known as the Centers for Medicare & Medicaid Services (CMS), to reform its certification and oversight of nursing homes for Medicare and Medicaid, which includes surveys to ensure the quality of resident care, complaint investigations, and remedies and penalties for nursing homes not in compliance with federal standards.[3]

The nation's 1.5 million nursing home residents are a highly vulnerable population of elderly and disabled individuals for whom remaining at home is no longer feasible. With the aging of the baby boom generation, the number of individuals needing nursing home care and the associated costs are expected to increase dramatically. Combined Medicare and Medicaid payments for nursing home services were about $72.7 billion in 2005, including a federal share of about $49 billion. The federal government plays a key role in ensuring that nursing home residents receive appropriate care by setting quality-of-care, quality-of-life, and life safety requirements that nursing homes must meet to participate in the Medicare and Medicaid programs and by contracting with states to routinely inspect homes and conduct complaint investigations.[4] To encourage compliance with these requirements, Congress has authorized certain enforcement actions.

Since this Committee requested us to investigate California nursing homes in 1997, we have reported to Congress and testified numerous times on the quality of resident care, identified significant weaknesses in federal and state activities designed to detect and correct quality problems in nursing homes, and made many recommendations to improve the survey process and federal oversight of nursing home quality.[5] In response to our recommendations as well as needed improvements CMS identified in its own self-assessment in 1998, CMS announced a set of initiatives intended to address many of these weaknesses. Over time, CMS has refined and expanded these initiatives in order to continue to improve nursing home quality.

My remarks today will focus on GAO's work in evaluating the quality of nursing home care and the enforcement and oversight functions intended to ensure high-quality care.[6] I will address the progress made in these three areas since OBRA '87, as well as the challenges that remain. This statement is based primarily on prior GAO work. In addition, we interviewed CMS officials; analyzed data from CMS's On-Line Survey, Certification, and Reporting system (OSCAR), which compiles the results of state nursing home surveys; and evaluated the results of federal comparative surveys for selected states for the period January 2005 through March 2007. Federal comparative surveys are conducted at nursing homes recently surveyed by each state to assess the adequacy of the state's surveys. We considered these data sufficiently reliable for our purposes. We discussed the highlights of this statement including our new analyses with CMS officials, and they provided us additional information, which we incorporated as appropriate. We conducted our work from March through April 2007 in accordance with generally accepted government auditing standards.

In summary, despite the reforms of OBRA '87 and subsequent efforts by CMS and the nursing home industry to improve the quality of nursing home care, a small but significant share of nursing homes nationwide continues to experience quality-of-care problems. In 2006, one in five nursing homes nationwide was cited for serious deficiencies—those deficiencies that cause actual harm or place residents in immediate jeopardy. While this rate has fluctuated over the last 7 years, we have regularly found (1) significant variation across states in their citation of serious deficiencies, indicating inconsistencies in states' assessments of quality of care and (2) understatement of these deficiencies—when deficiencies are found on federal comparative surveys but not cited on corresponding state surveys. Among the five large states we reviewed— California, Florida, New York, Ohio, and Texas—understatement of serious deficiencies has declined from 18 percent prior to December 2004 to 11 percent for the most recent time period ending in March 2007, but understatement has continued at varying levels.

Since the passage of OBRA '87, CMS has strengthened its enforcement capabilities—for example, by implementing sanctions authorized in the legislation, establishing an immediate sanctions policy for nursing homes found to repeatedly harm residents, and developing a new enforcement management data system—but several key initiatives require refinement. The immediate sanctions policy is complex and appears to have induced only temporary compliance in certain nursing homes with histories of repeated noncompliance. In addition, the term "immediate sanctions" policy is misleading because it requires only that homes be notified immediately of CMS's intent to implement sanctions, not that sanctions be implemented immediately. Furthermore, when a sanction, such as a denial of payment for new admissions (DPNA), is implemented, there is a lag time between when the deficiency citation occurs and the effective date of the sanction. Finally, although CMS has developed a new data system, the system's components are not integrated and the national reporting capabilities are incomplete, hampering the agency's ability to track and monitor enforcement.

CMS oversight of nursing home quality and state surveys has increased since OBRA '87, but certain key initiatives continue to compete for resources. To increase its oversight of quality of care in nursing homes, CMS has focused its resources and attention in areas such as prompt investigation of complaints and allegations of abuse, more frequent federal comparative surveys, stronger fire safety standards, and upgrades to data systems. However, this increased emphasis on nursing home oversight coupled with growth in the number of Medicare and Medicaid providers has caused greater demand on limited resources, which, in turn, has led to queues and delays in certain key initiatives. For example, the implementation of a new survey methodology, the Quality Indicator Survey (QIS), has been in development for over 8 years and resource constraints threaten the planned expansion of this methodology beyond the initial five demonstration states.

Significant attention from the Special Committee on Aging, the Institute of Medicine, and others served as a catalyst to focus national attention on nursing home quality issues, culminating in the nursing home reform provisions of OBRA '87. Since then, in response to many GAO recommendations and at its own initiative, CMS has taken many important steps to respond in a timelier, more rigorous, more consistent manner to identified problems. Nevertheless, the task of ensuring high-quality nursing home care is still not complete. To guarantee that all nursing home residents receive high-quality care, it is important to maintain the momentum begun by the reforms of OBRA '87 and continue to focus national attention on those homes that cause actual harm to vulnerable residents.

BACKGROUND

Titles XVIII and XIX of the Social Security Act establish minimum requirements that all nursing homes must meet to participate in the Medicare and Medicaid programs, respectively.

With the passage of OBRA '87, Congress responded to growing concerns about the quality of care that nursing home residents received by requiring major reforms in the federal regulation of nursing homes. Among other things, these reforms revised care requirements that facilities must meet to participate in the Medicare or Medicaid programs, modified the survey process for certifying a home's compliance with federal standards, and introduced additional sanctions and decertification procedures for homes that fail to meet federal standards. Following OBRA '87, CMS published a series of regulations and transmittals to implement the changes. Key implementation actions have included the following: In October 1990, CMS implemented new survey standards; in July 1995, it established enforcement actions for nursing homes found to be out of compliance; and it enhanced oversight through more rigorous federal monitoring surveys beginning in October 1998 and annual state performance reviews in fiscal year 2001. CMS has continued to revise and refine many of these actions since their initial implementation.

Survey Process

Every nursing home receiving Medicare or Medicaid payment must undergo a standard survey not less than once every 15 months, and the statewide average interval for these surveys must not exceed 12 months.[7] During a standard survey, separate teams of surveyors conduct a comprehensive assessment of federal quality-of-care and life safety requirements. In contrast, complaint investigations, also conducted by surveyors, generally focus on a specific allegation regarding resident care or safety.[8]

The quality-of-care component of a survey focuses on determining whether (1) the care and services provided meet the assessed needs of the residents and (2) the home is providing adequate quality care, including preventing avoidable pressure sores, weight loss, and accidents. Nursing homes that participate in Medicare and Medicaid are required to periodically assess residents' care needs in 17 areas, such as mood and behavior, physical functioning, and skin conditions, in order to develop an appropriate plan of care. Such resident assessment data are known as the minimum data set (MDS). To assess the care provided by a nursing home, surveyors select a sample of residents and (1) review data derived from the residents' MDS assessments and medical records; (2) interview nursing home staff, residents, and family members; and (3) observe care provided to residents during the course of the survey. CMS establishes specific investigative protocols for state survey teams—generally consisting of registered nurses, social workers, dieticians, and other specialists—to use in conducting surveys. These procedural instructions are intended to make the on-site surveys thorough and consistent across states.

The life safety component of a survey focuses on a home's compliance with federal fire safety requirements for health care facilities.[9] The fire safety requirements cover 18 categories, ranging from building construction to furnishings. Most states use fire safety specialists within the same department as the state survey agency to conduct fire safety inspections, but some states contract with their state fire marshal's office.

Complaint investigations provide an opportunity for state surveyors to intervene promptly if problems arise between standard surveys. Complaints may be filed against a home by a resident, the resident's family, or a nursing home employee either verbally, via a complaint hotline, or in writing. Surveyors generally follow state procedures when investigating complaints but must comply with certain federal guidelines and time frames. In cases involving resident abuse, such as pushing, slapping, beating, or otherwise assaulting a resident by individuals to whom their care has been entrusted, state survey agencies may notify state or local law enforcement agencies that can initiate criminal investigations. States must maintain a registry of qualified nurse aides, the primary caregivers in nursing homes, that includes any findings that an aide has been responsible for abuse, neglect, or theft of a resident's property. The inclusion of such a finding constitutes a ban on nursing home employment.

Effective July 1995, CMS established a classification system for deficiencies identified during either standard surveys or complaint investigations. Deficiencies are classified in 1 of 12 categories according to their scope (i.e., the number of residents potentially or actually affected) and their severity. An A-level deficiency is the least serious and is isolated in scope, while an L-level deficiency is the most serious and is considered to be widespread in the nursing home (see table 1). States are required to enter information about surveys and complaint investigations, including the scope and severity of deficiencies identified, in CMS's OSCAR database.

Enforcement

In an effort to better ensure that nursing homes achieve and maintain compliance with the new survey standards, OBRA '87 expanded the range of enforcement sanctions. Prior to OBRA '87, the only sanctions available were terminations from Medicare or Medicaid or, under certain circumstances, DPNAs. OBRA '87 added several new alternative sanctions, such as civil money penalties (CMP) and requiring training for staff providing care to residents, and expanded the types of deficiencies that could result in DPNAs. To implement OBRA '87, CMS published enforcement regulations, effective July 1995. According to these regulations, the scope and severity of a deficiency determine the applicable sanctions. CMS imposes sanctions on homes with Medicare or dual Medicare and Medicaid certification on the basis of state referrals.[10] CMS normally accepts a state's recommendation for sanctions but can modify it.

Table 1. Scope and Severity of Deficiencies Identified during Nursing Home Surveys

	Scope		
Severity	**Isolated**	**Pattern**	**Widespread**
Immediate jeopardy[a]	J	K	L
Actual harm	G	H	I
Potential for more than minimal harm	D	E	F
Potential for minimal harm[b]	A	B	C

Source: CMS.

[a]Actual or potential for death/serious injury.

[b]Nursing home is considered to be in "substantial compliance."

Effective January 2000, CMS required states to refer for immediate sanction homes found to have harmed one or a small number of residents or to have a pattern of harming or exposing residents to actual harm or potential death or serious injury (G-level or higher deficiencies on the agency's scope and severity grid) on successive surveys. This is known as the double G immediate sanctions policy. Additionally, in January 1999, CMS launched the Special Focus Facility program. This initiative was intended to increase the oversight of homes with a history of providing poor care. When CMS established this program, it instructed each state to select two homes for enhanced monitoring. For these homes, states are to conduct surveys at 6-month intervals rather than annually. In December 2004, CMS expanded this program to require immediate sanctions for those homes that fail to significantly improve their performance from one survey to the next and termination for homes with no significant improvement after three surveys over an 18-month period.[11]

Unlike other sanctions, CMPs do not require a notification period before they go into effect. However, if a nursing home appeals the deficiency, by statute, payment of the CMP—whether received directly from the home or withheld from the home's Medicare and Medicaid payments—is deferred until the appeal is resolved.[12] In contrast to CMPs, other sanctions, including DPNAs, cannot go into effect until homes have been provided a notice period of at least 15 days, according to CMS regulations; the notice period is shortened to 2 days in the case of immediate jeopardy. Although nursing homes can be terminated involuntarily from participation in Medicare and Medicaid, which can result in a home's closure, termination is used infrequently.[13]

Oversight

CMS is responsible for overseeing each state survey agency's performance in ensuring quality of care in nursing homes participating in Medicare or Medicaid. Its primary oversight tools are (1) statutorily required federal monitoring surveys and (2) annual state performance reviews. Pursuant to OBRA '87, CMS is required to conduct annual monitoring surveys in at least 5 percent of the state-surveyed Medicare and Medicaid nursing homes in each state, with a minimum of five facilities in each state. These federal monitoring surveys can be either comparative or observational. A comparative survey involves a federal survey team conducting a complete, independent survey of a home within 2 months of the completion of a state's survey in order to compare and contrast the findings. In an observational survey, one or more federal surveyors accompany a state survey team to a nursing home to observe the team's performance. State performance reviews measure state survey agency compliance with seven standards: timeliness of the survey, documentation of survey results, quality of state agency investigations and decision making, timeliness of enforcement actions, budget analysis, timeliness and quality of complaint investigations, and timeliness and accuracy of data entry. These reviews replaced state self-reporting of their compliance with federal requirements.

Quality of Care Remains a Problem for a Small but Significant Proportion of Nursing Homes Nationwide

A small but significant proportion of nursing homes nationwide continue to experience quality-of-care problems—as evidenced by the almost 1 in 5 nursing homes nationwide that were cited for serious deficiencies in 2006—despite the reforms of OBRA '87 and subsequent efforts by CMS and the nursing home industry to improve the quality of nursing home care. Although there has been an overall decline in the numbers of nursing homes found to have serious deficiencies since fiscal year 2000, variation among states in the proportion of homes with serious deficiencies indicates state survey agencies are not consistently conducting surveys. Challenges associated with the recruitment and retention of state surveyors, combined with increased surveyor workloads, can affect survey consistency. In addition, federal comparative surveys conducted after state surveys found more serious quality-of-care problems than were cited by state surveyors. Although understatement of serious deficiencies identified by federal surveyors in five states has declined since 2004, understatement continues at varying levels across these states.

CMS data indicate an overall decline in reported serious deficiencies from fiscal year 2000 through 2006. The proportion of nursing homes nationwide cited with serious deficiencies declined from 28 percent in fiscal year 2000 to a low of 16 percent in 2004, and then increased to 19 percent in fiscal year 2006 (see figure 1).

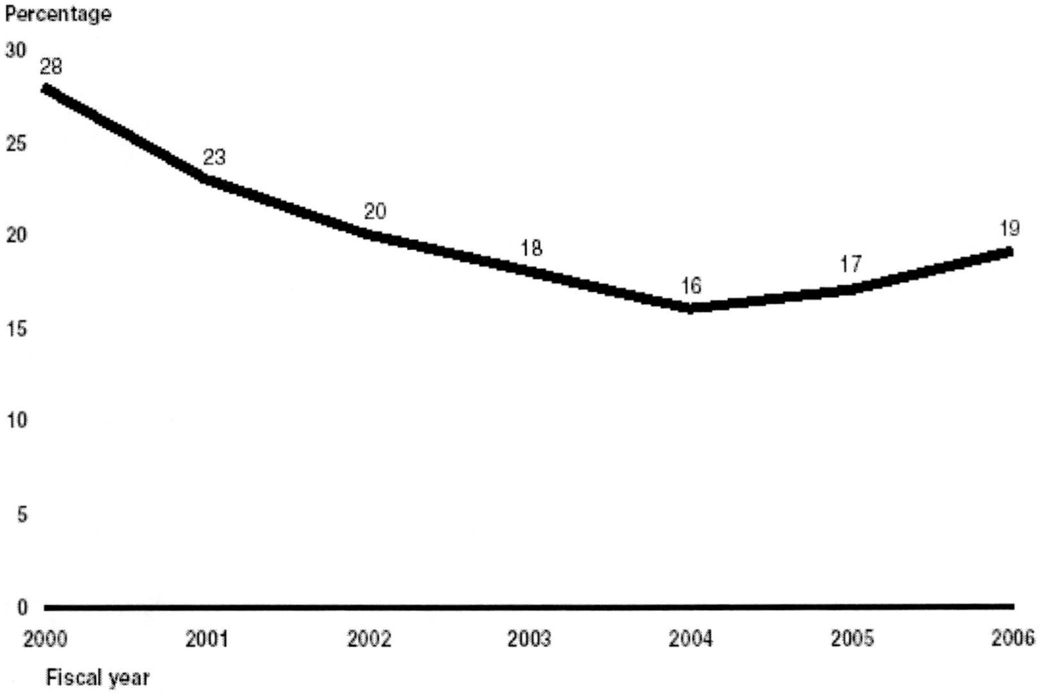

Source: GAO analysis of OSCAR data.

Figure 1. Percentage of Nursing Homes Nationwide with Serious Deficiencies, Fiscal Years 2000-2006

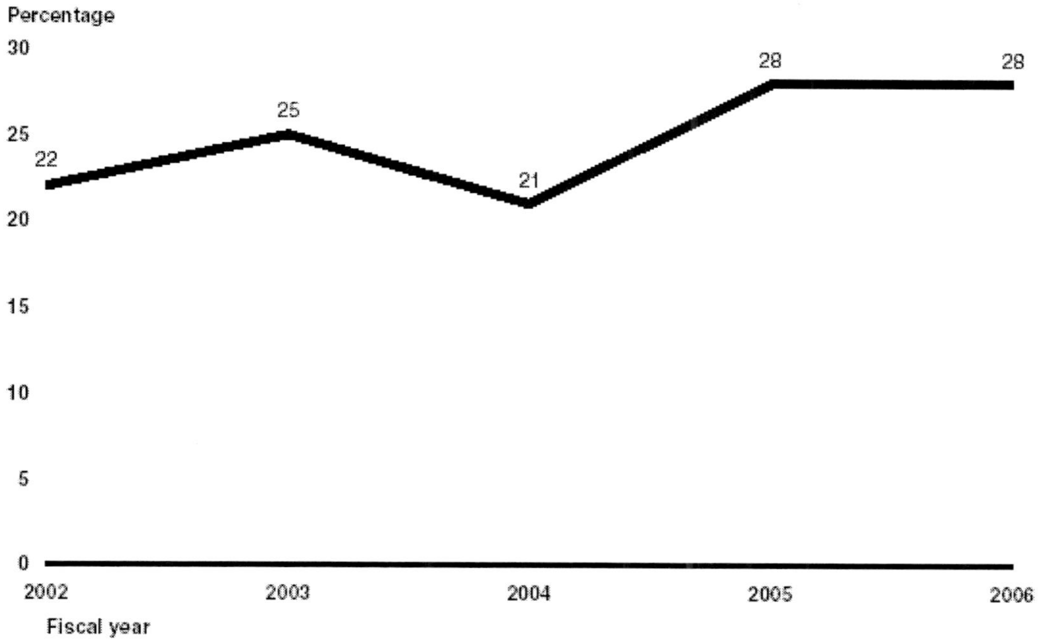

Source: GAO analysis of OSCAR data.

Figure 2. Percentage of Federal Comparative Surveys That Noted Serious Deficiencies Not Identified in State Surveys

Despite this national trend, significant interstate variation in the proportion of homes with serious deficiencies indicates that states conduct surveys inconsistently. (App. II shows the percentage of homes, by state, cited for serious deficiencies in standard surveys across a 7-year period.). In fiscal year 2006, 6 states identified serious deficiencies in 30 percent or more of homes surveyed, 16 states found such deficiencies in 20 to 30 percent of homes, 22 found these deficiencies in 10 to 19 percent of homes, and 7 found these deficiencies in less than 10 percent of homes. For example, in fiscal year 2006, the percentage of nursing homes cited for serious deficiencies ranged from a low of approximately 2 percent in one state to a high of almost 51 percent in another state.

The inconsistency of state survey findings may reflect challenges in recruiting and retaining state surveyors and increasing state surveyor workloads. We reported in 2005 that, according to state survey agency officials, it is difficult to retain surveyors and fill vacancies because state survey agency salaries are rarely competitive with the private sector.[14] Moreover, the first year for a new surveyor is essentially a training period with low productivity. It can take as long as 3 years for a surveyor to gain sufficient knowledge, experience, and confidence to perform the job well. We also reported that limited experience levels of state surveyors resulting from high turnover rates was a contributing factor to (1) variability in citing actual harm or higher-level deficiencies and (2) understatement of such deficiencies. In addition, the implementation of CMS's nursing home initiatives has increased state survey agencies' workload. States are now required to conduct on-site revisits to ensure serious deficiencies have been corrected, promptly investigate complaints alleging actual harm on- site, and initiate off-hour standard surveys in addition to quality-of-care surveys. As a result, surveyor presence in nursing homes has increased and surveyor work hours have effectively been expanded to weekends, evenings, and early mornings.

In addition, data from federal comparative surveys indicate that quality-of-care problems remain for a significant proportion of nursing homes. In fiscal year 2006, 28 percent of federal comparative surveys found more serious deficiencies than did state quality-of-care surveys. Since 2002, federal surveyors have found serious deficiencies in 21 percent or more of comparative surveys that were not cited in corresponding state quality-ofcare surveys (see figure 2). However, some serious deficiencies found by federal, but not state surveyors, may not have existed at the time the state survey occurred.[15]

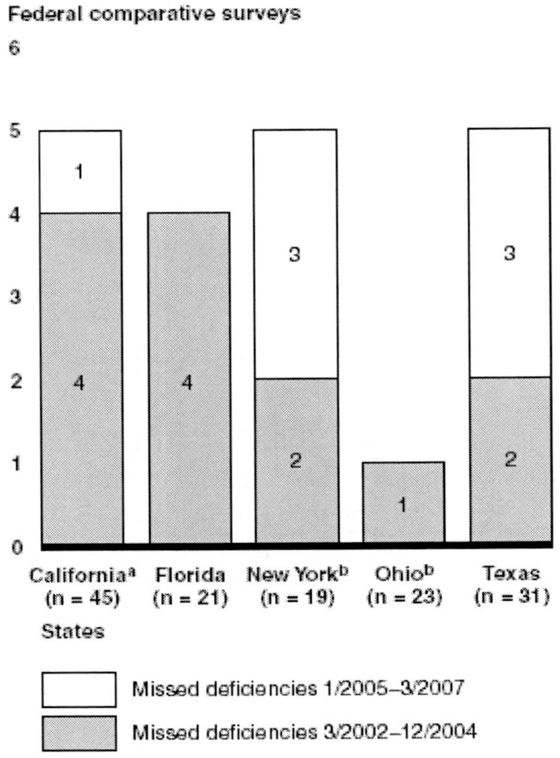

Source: GAO analysis of federal comparative surveys for five years.

Notes: The total number of federal comparative surveys conducted in each state for the 5-year period, March 2002 to March 2007, is listed in parentheses following the name of the state. The percentage of federal comparative surveys that noted serious deficiencies missed by state surveyors in each state was California, 11 percent; Florida, 19 percent; New York, 26 percent; Ohio, 4 percent; and Texas, 16 percent.

[a] On two comparative surveys, federal surveyors did not provide information on whether any of the deficiencies they identified existed at the time of the state survey; therefore, this number may be understated.

[b] On one comparative survey, federal surveyors did not provide information on whether any of the deficiencies they identified existed at the time of the state survey; therefore, this number may be understated.

Figure 3. Federal Comparative Surveys in Five States That Identified Serious Deficiencies Missed by State Surveys, March 2002-March 2007

In December 2005, we reported on understatement of serious deficiencies in five states—California, Florida, New York, Ohio, and Texas—from March 2002 through December 2004.[16] We selected these states for our analysis because the percentage of their state surveys that cited serious deficiencies decreased significantly from January 1999 through January 2005.[17] Our analysis of more recent data from these states showed that understatement of serious deficiencies continues at varying levels. Altogether, we examined 139 federal comparative surveys conducted from March 2002 through March 2007 in the five states. Understatement of serious deficiencies decreased from 18 percent for federal comparative surveys during the original time period to 11 percent for federal comparative surveys during the period January 2005 through March 2007.

Federal comparative surveys for Florida and Ohio for this most recent time period found that state surveys had not missed any serious deficiencies; however, since 2004 all five states experienced increases in the percentage of homes cited with serious deficiencies on state surveys (see app. II). Understatement of serious deficiencies varied across these five states, as the percentage of serious missed deficiencies ranged from a low of 4 percent in Ohio to a high of 26 percent in New York during the 5- year period March 2002 to March 2007. Figure 3 summarizes our analysis by state, from March 2002 through March 2007.

CMS Has Strengthened Its Enforcement Capabilities, although Key Initiatives Still Need Refinement

CMS has strengthened its enforcement capabilities since OBRA ‘87 by, for example, implementing additional sanctions and an immediate sanctions policy for nursing homes found to repeatedly harm residents and developing a new enforcement management data system; however, several key initiatives require refinement. The immediate sanctions policy is complex and appears to have induced only temporary compliance in certain nursing homes with histories of repeated noncompliance. The term “immediate sanctions” is misleading because the policy requires only that homes be notified immediately of CMS’s intent to implement sanctions, not that sanctions must be implemented immediately. Furthermore, when a sanction is implemented, there is a lag time between when the deficiency citation occurs and the sanction’s effective date. In addition to the immediate sanctions policy, CMS has taken other steps that are intended to address enforcement weaknesses, but their effectiveness remains unclear. Finally, although CMS has developed a new data system, the system’s components are not integrated and the national reporting capabilities are incomplete, hampering the agency’s ability to track and monitor enforcement.

Despite Changes in Federal Enforcement Policy, Immediate Sanctions Do Not Always Deter Noncompliance and Often Are Not Immediate

Despite CMS’s efforts to strengthen federal enforcement policy, it has not deterred some homes from repeatedly harming residents. Effective January 2000, CMS implemented its double G immediate sanctions policy. The policy is complex and does not always appear to deter noncompliance, nor are the sanctions always implemented immediately. We recently reported that the immediate sanctions policy's complex rules, and the exceptions they include, allowed homes to escape immediate sanctions even if they repeatedly harmed residents.[18] CMS acknowledged that the complexity of the policy may be an inherent limitation and indicated that it intends to either strengthen the policy or replace it with a policy that achieves similar goals through alternative methods.

In addition to the complexity of the policy, it does not appear to always deter noncompliance. We recently reported that our review of 63 homes with prior serious quality problems in four states indicated that sanctions may have induced only temporary compliance in these homes because surveyors found that many of the homes with implemented sanctions were again out of compliance on subsequent surveys.[19] From fiscal year 2000 through 2005, 31 of these 63 homes cycled in and out of compliance more than once, harming residents, even after sanctions had been implemented, including 8 homes that did so seven times or more. During this same time period, 27 of the 63 homes were cited 69 times for deficiencies that warranted immediate sanctions, but 15 of these cases did not result in immediate sanctions.[20]

We also recently reported that the term "immediate sanctions" is misleading because the policy is silent on how quickly sanctions should be implemented and there is a lag time between the state's identification of deficiencies during the survey and when the sanction (i.e., a CMP or DPNA) is implemented (i.e., when it goes into effect). The immediate sanctions policy requires that sanctions be imposed immediately. A sanction is considered imposed when a home is notified of CMS's intent to implement a sanction—15 days from the date of the notice. If during the 15-day notice period the nursing home corrects the deficiencies, no sanction is implemented. Thus, nursing homes have a de facto grace period. In addition, there is a lag time between the state's identification of deficiencies and the implementation of a sanction. CMS implemented about 68 percent of the DPNAs for double Gs among the homes we reviewed during fiscal year 2000 through 2005 more than 30 days after the survey.[21] In contrast, CMPs can go into effect as early as the first day the home was out of compliance, even if that date is prior to the survey date because, unlike DPNAs, CMPs do not require a notice period. About 98 percent of CMPs imposed for double Gs took effect on or before the survey date. However, the deterrent effect of CMPs was diluted because CMS imposed CMPs at the lower end of the allowable range for the homes we reviewed. For example, the median per day CMP amount imposed for deficiencies that do not cause immediate jeopardy to residents was $500 in fiscal year 2000 through 2002 and $350 in fiscal year 2003 through 2005; the allowable range is $50 to $3,000 per day.

Although CMPs can be implemented closer to the date of survey than DPNAs, the immediacy and the effect of CMPs may be diminished by (1) the significant time that can pass between the citation of deficiencies on a survey and the home's payment of the CMP and (2) the low amounts imposed, as described earlier. By statute, payment of CMPs is delayed until appeals are exhausted. For example, one home we reviewed did not pay its CMP of $21,600 until more than 2 years after a February 2003 survey had cited a G-level deficiency. This citation was a repeat deficiency: less than a month earlier, the home had received another G-level deficiency in the same quality-of-care area. This finding is consistent with a 2005 report from the Department of Health and Human Services' (HHS) Office of Inspector General that found that the collection of CMPs in appealed cases takes an average of 420 days—a 110 percent increase in time over nonappealed cases—and "consequently, nursing homes are insulated from the repercussions of enforcement by well over a year."[22]

CMS has taken additional steps intended to improve enforcement of nursing home quality requirements; however, the extent to which—or when—these initiatives will address enforcement weaknesses remains unclear. First, to ensure greater consistency in CMP amounts proposed by states and imposed by regions, CMS, in conjunction with state survey agencies, developed a grid that provides guidance for states and regions. The CMP grid lists ranges for minimum CMP amounts while allowing for flexibility to adjust the penalties for factors such as the deficiency's scope and severity, the care areas where the deficiency was cited, and a home's past history of noncompliance. In August 2006, CMS completed the regional office pilot of its CMP grid but had not completed its analysis of the pilot as of April 2007. CMS plans to disseminate the final grid to states soon.[23] Second, in December 2004, CMS expanded the Special Focus Facility program from about 100 homes to include about 135 homes. CMS also modified the program by requiring immediate sanctions for those homes that failed to significantly improve their performance from one survey to the next and by requiring termination for homes with no significant improvement after three surveys over an 18-month period. According to CMS, 11 Special Focus Facilities were terminated in fiscal year 2005 and 7 were terminated in fiscal year 2006. Despite the expansion of the program, many homes that could benefit from enhanced oversight and enforcement are still excluded from the program. For example, of the 63 homes with prior serious quality problems that we recently reviewed, only 2 were designated Special Focus Facilities in 2005, and the number increased to 4 in 2006.

While CMS Collects Valuable Enforcement Data, Its Enforcement Monitoring Data Systems Need Improvement

In March 1999, we reported that CMS lacked a system for effectively integrating enforcement data nationwide and that the lack of such a system weakened oversight. Since 1999, CMS has made progress developing such a system—ASPEN Enforcement Manager (AEM)—and, since October 1, 2004, CMS has used AEM to collect state and regional data on sanctions and improve communications between state survey agencies and CMS regional offices. CMS expects that the data collected in AEM will enable states, CMS regional offices, and the CMS central office to more easily track and evaluate sanctions against nursing homes as well as respond to emerging issues. Developed by CMS's central office primarily for use by states and regions, AEM is one of many modules of a broader data collection system called ASPEN. However, the ASPEN modules—and other data systems related to enforcement such as the financial management system for tracking CMP collections—are fragmented and lack automated interfaces with each other. As a result, enforcement officials must pull discrete bits of data from the various systems and manually combine the data to develop a full enforcement picture.

Furthermore, CMS has not defined a plan for using the AEM data to inform the tracking and monitoring of enforcement through national enforcement reports. While CMS is developing a few such reports, it has not developed a concrete plan and timeline for producing a full set of reports that use the AEM data to help assess the effectiveness of sanctions and its enforcement policies. In addition, while the full complement of enforcement data being recorded by the states and regional offices in AEM is now being uploaded to

CMS's national system, CMS does not intend to upload any historical data, which could greatly enhance enforcement monitoring efforts. Finally, AEM has quality control weaknesses, such as the lack of systematic quality control mechanisms to ensure accuracy of data entry.

CMS officials told us they will continue to develop and implement enhancements to AEM to expand its capabilities over the next several years. However, until CMS develops a plan for integrating the fragmented systems and for using AEM data—along with other data the agency collects—efficient and effective tracking and monitoring of enforcement will continue to be hampered. As a result, CMS will have difficulty assessing the effectiveness of sanctions and its enforcement policies.[24]

CMS Has Strengthened Oversight, although Competing Priorities Impede Certain Key Initiatives

CMS oversight of nursing home quality and state surveys has increased significantly through several efforts, but CMS initiatives for nursing home quality oversight continue to compete with each other, as well as with other CMS programs, for staff and financial resources. Since OBRA '87 required CMS to annually conduct federal monitoring surveys for a sample of nursing homes to test the adequacy of state surveys, CMS has developed a number of initiatives to strengthen its oversight. These initiatives have increased federal surveyors' workload and the demand for resources. Greater demand on limited resources has led to queues and delays in certain key initiatives. In particular, the implementation of three key initiatives—the new Quality Indicator Survey (QIS), investigative protocols for quality-of-care problems, and an increase in the number of federal quality-of-care comparative surveys—was delayed because they compete for priority with other CMS projects.

Intensity of Federal Efforts Has Increased Significantly

CMS has used both federal monitoring surveys and annual state performance reviews to increase its oversight of quality of care in nursing homes. Through these two mechanisms it has focused its resources and attention on (1) prompt investigation of complaints and allegations of abuse, (2) more frequent and timely federal comparative surveys, (3) stronger fire safety standards, and (4) upgrades to data systems.

Complaint investigations

To ensure that complaints and allegations of abuse are investigated and addressed in accordance with OBRA '87, CMS has issued guidance and taken other steps. CMS guidance issued since 1999 has helped strengthen state procedures for investigating complaints. For example, CMS instructed states to investigate complaints alleging harm to a resident within 10 workdays; previously states could establish their own time frames for complaints at this level of severity. In addition, CMS guidance to states in 2002 and 2004 clarified policies on reporting abuse, including requiring notification of local law enforcement and Medicaid Fraud Control Units, establishing time frames, and citing abuse on surveys.

CMS has taken three additional steps to improve its oversight of state complaint investigations, including allegations of abuse. First, in its annual state performance reviews implemented in 2002, it required that federal surveyors review a sample of complaints in each state.[25] These reviews were done to determine whether states (1) properly categorized complaints in terms of how quickly they should be investigated, (2) investigated complaints within the time specified, and (3) properly included the results of the investigations in CMS's database. Second, in January 2004, CMS implemented a new national automated complaint tracking system, the ASPEN Complaints and Incidents Tracking System. The lack of a national complaint reporting system had hindered CMS's and states' ability to adequately track the status of complaint investigations and CMS's ability to maintain a full compliance history on each nursing home. Third, in November 2004, CMS requested state survey agency directors to self-assess their states' compliance with federal requirements for maintaining and operating nurse aide registries. CMS has not issued a formal report of findings from these assessments, but in 2005 we reported that CMS officials noted that resource constraints have impeded states' compliance with certain federal requirements.[26] As a part of this effort, CMS is also conducting a Background Check Pilot Program. The pilot program will test the effectiveness of state and national fingerprint-based background checks on employees of long-term care facilities, including nursing homes.[27]

Federal Comparative Surveys

CMS has increased the number of federal comparative surveys for both quality of care and fire safety and decreased the time between the end of the state survey and the start of the federal comparative surveys. These improvements allow CMS to better distinguish between serious problems missed by state surveyors and changes in the home that occurred after the state survey. The number of comparative quality-of-care surveys nationwide per year increased from about 10 surveys a year during the 24-month period prior to October 1998 to about 160 per year for fiscal years 2005 and 2006.[28] The number of fire safety comparative surveys increased as well from 40 in fiscal year 2003 to 536 in fiscal year 2006. In addition, the average elapsed time between state and comparative qualityof-care surveys has decreased from 33 calendar days for the 64 comparative surveys we reviewed in 1999 to 26 days for all federal comparative surveys completed through fiscal year 2006.

Fire Safety Standards

In addition to conducting more frequent federal comparative surveys for fire safety, CMS has strengthened fire safety standards. In response to a recommendation in our July 2004 report to strengthen fire safety standards,[29] CMS issued a final rule in September 2006 requiring nonsprinklered nursing homes to install battery-powered smoke detectors in resident rooms and common areas.[30] In addition, CMS has issued a proposed rule that would require all nursing homes to be equipped with sprinkler systems and, after reviewing public comment, intends to publish a final version of the rule and stipulate an effective date for all homes to comply.[31]

Upgrades to Data Systems

CMS has pursued important upgrades to data systems, expanded dissemination of data and information, and addressed accuracy issues in the MDS in addition to implementing complaint and enforcement systems. One such upgrade increased state and federal surveyors' access to OSCAR data. CMS now uses OSCAR data to produce periodic reports to monitor both state and federal survey performance. Some reports, such as survey timeliness, are used during state performance reviews, while others are intended to help identify problems or inconsistencies in state survey activities and the need for intervention. In addition, CMS created a Web- accessible software program called Providing Data Quickly (PDQ) that allows regional offices and state survey agencies easier access to standard OSCAR reports, including one that identifies the homes that have repeatedly harmed residents and meet the criteria for imposition of immediate sanctions.

Since launching its Nursing Home Compare Web site in 1998, CMS has expanded its dissemination of information to the public on individual nursing homes participating in Medicare or Medicaid.[32] In addition to data on any deficiencies identified during standard surveys, the Web site now includes data on the results of complaint investigations, information on nursing home staffing levels, and quality measures, such as the percentage of residents with pressure sores. On the basis of our recommendations, CMS is now reporting fire safety deficiencies on the Web site, including information on whether a home has automatic sprinklers to suppress a fire, and may include information on impending sanctions in the future. However, CMS continues to address ongoing problems with the accuracy and reliability of some of the underlying data. For example, CMS has evaluated the validity of quality measures and staffing information it makes available on the Web, and it has removed or excluded questionable data.

In addition to building the quality measures reported on Nursing Home Compare, the MDS data are the basis for patient care plans, adjusting Medicare nursing home payments as well as Medicaid payments in some states, and assisting with quality oversight. Thus the accuracy of the MDS has implications for the identification of quality problems and the level of nursing home payments. OBRA '87 required nursing homes that participate in the Medicare and Medicaid programs to perform periodic resident assessments; these resident assessments are known as the MDS. In February 2002, we assessed federal government efforts to ensure the accuracy of the MDS data.[33] We reported that on-site reviews of MDS data that compared the MDS to supporting documentation were a very effective method of assessing the accuracy of the data. However, CMS's efforts to ensure the accuracy of the underlying MDS data were too reliant on off- site reviews, which were limited to documentation reviews or data analysis. To ensure the accuracy of the MDS, CMS signed a new contract for on-site reviews in September 2005; these reviews are ongoing.

Competing Priorities Impede Certain Key CMS Initiatives

CMS initiatives for nursing home quality oversight continue to compete with each other, as well as with other CMS programs, for staff and financial resources. Greater nursing home oversight and growth in the number of Medicare and Medicaid providers has created increased demand for staff and financial resources. Greater demand on limited resources has led to queues and delays in key initiatives. Three key initiatives—the new Quality Indicator Survey (QIS), investigative protocols for quality-of-care problems, and an increase in the number of federal quality-of-care comparative surveys—were delayed because they compete for priority with other CMS projects.

The implementation of the QIS, in process for over 8 years, continues to encounter delays because of a lack of resources. The QIS is a two-stage, data-driven, structured survey process intended to systematically target potential problems at nursing homes by using an expanded sample and structured interviews to help surveyors better assess the scope of any identified deficiencies. CMS is currently concluding a five-state demonstration of the QIS system. A preliminary evaluation by CMS indicates that surveyors have spent less time in homes that are performing well, deficiency citations were linked to more defensible documentation, and serious deficiencies were more frequently cited in some demonstration states. However, CMS officials recently reported that resource constraints in fiscal year 2007 threaten the planned expansion of this process beyond the five demonstration states. Although 13 states applied to transition to QIS, resource limitations may prevent this expansion. In addition, at least $2 million is needed over 2 years to develop a production quality software package for the QIS.

Since hiring a contractor in 2001 to facilitate convening expert panels for the development and review of new investigative protocols, CMS has implemented eight sets of investigative protocols. In December 2005, we reported that these investigative protocols provided surveyors with detailed interpretive guidance and ensured greater rigor in on-site investigations of specific quality-of-care areas, such as pressure sores, incontinence, and medical director qualifications. However, the issuance of additional protocols was slowed because of lengthy consultation with experts and prolonged delays related to internal disagreement over the structure of the process. Instead, it has returned to the traditional revision process even though agency staff believes that the expert panel process produced a high-quality product. Since issuing several protocols in 2006, CMS has plans to issue two additional protocols.

Although CMS hired a contractor in 2003 to further increase the number of federal quality-of-care comparative surveys, it stopped funding this initiative in fiscal year 2006. The agency reallocated the funds to help state survey agencies meet the increased workload resulting from growth in the number of other Medicare providers.

Concluding Observations

About 20 years ago, significant attention from the Special Committee on Aging, the Institute of Medicine, and others served as a catalyst to focus national attention on nursing home quality issues, culminating in the nursing home reform provisions of OBRA '87. Beginning in 1998, the Committee again served as a catalyst to focus national attention on the fact that the task was not complete; through a series of hearings, it held the various stakeholders publicly accountable for the substandard care reported in a small but significant share of nursing homes nationwide. Since then, in response to many GAO recommendations and on its own initiative, CMS has taken many important steps and invested resources to respond in a timelier, more rigorous, and more consistent manner to identified problems and improve its oversight process for the care of vulnerable nursing home residents. This is admittedly no small undertaking, given the large number and diversity of stakeholders and caregivers involved at the federal, state, and provider levels. Nevertheless, despite the passage of time and the level of investment and effort, the work begun after OBRA '87 is still not complete. It is important to continue to focus national attention on and ensure public accountability for homes that harm residents. With these ongoing efforts, the momentum of earlier initiatives can be sustained and perhaps even enhanced and the quality of care for nursing home residents can be secured, as intended by Congress when it passed this legislation.

Mr. Chairman, this concludes my prepared remarks. I would be pleased to respond to any questions that you or other Members of the Committee may have.

Appendix I. Prior GAO Recommendations, Related CMS Initiatives, and Implementation Status

Table 2. Implementation Status of CMS's Initiatives Responding to GAO's Nursing Home Quality and Safety Recommendations, July 1998 through April 2007

GAO report number	GAO recommendation	CMS initiative	Implementation status
Surveys			
GAO/HEHS-98-202	1. Stagger or otherwise vary the scheduling of standard surveys to effectively reduce the predictability of surveyors' visits. The variation could include segmenting the standard survey into more than one review throughout the 12- to 15-month period, which would provide more opportunities for surveyors to observe problematic homes and initiate broader reviews when warranted.	CMS took several steps to reduce survey predictability, but some state surveys remain predictable. • In 1999, CMS instructed state survey agencies to (1) conduct 10 percent of surveys on evenings and weekends, (2) vary the sequencing of surveys in a geographical area to avoid alerting other homes that the surveyors are in the area, (3) vary the scheduling of surveys by day of the week, and (4) avoid scheduling surveys for the same month as a home's prior survey. • In 2004, CMS provided states with an automated scheduling and tracking system (AST) to assist in scheduling surveys. CMS officials told us that AST can be used to address survey predictability. States appeared to be unaware of this feature and use of AST is optional. • CMS disagreed with and did not implement the recommendation to segment the standard survey into more than one review throughout the 12- to 15-month period.	◑
	2. Revise federal survey procedures to instruct surveyors to take stratified random samples of resident cases and review sufficient numbers and types	CMS has been developing a revised survey methodology since 1998. A pilot test of the new	○

Table 2. (Continued)

GAO report number	GAO recommendation	CMS initiative	Implementation status
	of resident cases so that surveyors can better detect problems and assess their prevalence.	methodology began in the fall of 2005. Implementation could begin in mid-2007.	
GAO-03-561	3. Finalize the development, testing, and implementation of a more rigorous survey methodology, including investigative protocols that provide guidance to surveyors in documenting deficiencies at the appropriate scope and severity level.	See CMS action in response to recommendation to revise federal survey procedures (recommendation #2 above). CMS began revising surveyors' investigative protocols in October 2000. Eight protocols have been issued, and two additional protocols are under development. Due to issues with interpretation, CMS is no longer planning to issue definitions of actual harm and immediate jeopardy outside of the regulations.	○
	4. Require states to have a quality assurance process that includes, at a minimum, a review of a sample of survey reports below the level of actual harm to assess the appropriateness of the scope and severity cited and to help reduce instances of understated quality-of-care problems.	CMS has no plans to implement this recommendation, indicating that regular workload and priorities take precedence over it.	⊗
GAO-05-78	5. Hold homes accountable for all past noncompliance resulting in harm to residents, not just care problems deemed to be egregious, and develop an approach for citing such past noncompliance in a manner that clearly identifies the specific nature of the care problem both in the OSCAR database and on CMS's Nursing Home Compare Web site.	CMS revised its definition of past noncompliance. While CMS has not ruled out placing enforcement information on its Nursing Home Compare Web site in the future, CMS officials told us that resource constraints limit the agency's ability to do so at the current time.	○
Complaints			
GAO/HEHS-99-80	6. Develop additional standards for the prompt investigation of serious complaints alleging situations that may harm residents but are categorized as less than immediate jeopardy. These standards should include maximum allowable time frames for investigating serious complaints and for complaints that may be deferred until the next scheduled annual survey. States may continue to set priority levels and time frames that are more stringent than these federal standards.	In October 1999, CMS issued a policy letter stating that complaints alleging harm must be investigated within 10 days. In January 2004, CMS provided detailed direction and guidance to states for managing complaint investigations for numerous types of providers, including nursing homes. In June 2004, CMS made available updated guidance on the Internet that consolidates complaint investigation procedures for numerous types of providers.	●
	7. Strengthen federal oversight of state complaint investigations, including monitoring states' practices regarding priority-setting, on-site investigation, and timely reporting of serious health and safety complaints.	In 2000, CMS began requiring its regional offices to perform yearly assessments of states' complaint investigations as part of annual state performance reviews.	●

Table 2. (Continued)

GAO report number	GAO recommendation	CMS initiative	Implementation status
GAO-03-561	8. Finalize the development of guidance to states for their complaint investigation processes and ensure that it addresses key weaknesses, including the prioritization of	In January 2004, CMS provided detailed direction and guidance to states for managing complaint investigations for numerous types of providers, including nursing homes.	
	complaints for investigation, particularly those alleging harm to residents; the handling of facility self-reported incidents; and the use of appropriate complaint investigation practices.	In June 2004, CMS made available updated guidance on the Internet that consolidates complaint investigation procedures for numerous types of providers.	●
GAO-02-312	9. Ensure that state survey agencies immediately notify local law enforcement agencies or Medicaid Fraud Control Units when nursing homes report allegations of resident physical or sexual abuse or when the survey agency has confirmed complaints of alleged abuse.	In 2002, CMS issued a memorandum to the regional offices and state survey agencies emphasizing its policy for preventing abuse in nursing homes and for promptly reporting it to the appropriate agencies when it occurs. CMS determined it does not have the legal authority to require state survey agencies to report suspected physical and sexual abuse of nursing home residents.	◑
	10. Accelerate the agency's education campaign on reporting nursing home abuse by (1) distributing its new poster with clearly displayed complaint telephone numbers and (2) requiring state survey agencies to ensure that these numbers are prominently listed in local telephone directories.	In 2002, CMS released a memorandum to regional offices and state agencies that addresses displaying complaint telephone numbers. CMS asked all state agencies to review how their telephone number is listed in the local directory and asked them to ensure that their complaint telephone numbers are prominently listed. In 2007, CMS officials told us that it has not and is not likely to release the poster.	◑
	11. Systematically assess state policies and practices for complying with the federal requirement to prohibit employment of individuals convicted of abusing nursing home residents and, if necessary, develop more specific guidance to ensure compliance.	CMS is conducting a Background Check Pilot Program in several states, as required by the Medicare Prescription Drug, Improvement, and Modernization Act of 2003. The pilot is expected to run through September 2007 and will be followed by an independent evaluation. The final study is targeted for submission by spring of 2008.	○
	12. Clarify the definition of abuse and otherwise ensure that states apply that definition consistently and appropriately.	In 2002, CMS released a memorandum to its regional offices and state survey agency directors clarifying its definition of abuse and instructing them to report suspected abuse to law enforcement authorities and, if appropriate, to the state's Medicaid Fraud Control Unit.[a]	●

Table 2. (Continued)

GAO report number	GAO recommendation	CMS initiative	Implementation status
	13. Shorten the state survey agencies' time frames for determining whether to include findings of abuse in nurse aide registry files.	CMS informed GAO that federal regulations specify that if an investigation finds an individual has neglected or abused a resident or misappropriated resident property, the state must report the findings in writing within 10 working days to the nurse aide registry.	
		However, CMS stated it does not specify a time frame for completion of such investigations due to concerns that a time limit could compromise complaint investigations in some instances.	◑
Enforcement			
GAO/HEHS-98-202	14. Require that for problem homes with recurring serious violations, state surveyors substantiate, by means of an on-site revisit, every report to CMS of a home's resumed compliance status.	In 1998, CMS issued guidance to regional offices and state survey agencies strengthening its revisit policy by requiring on-site revisits until all serious deficiencies are corrected. Homes are no longer permitted to self-report resumed compliance.	●
	15. Eliminate the grace period for homes cited for repeated serious violations and impose sanctions promptly, as permitted under existing regulations.	CMS phased in implementation of its double G policy from September 1998 through January 2000.	●
GAO/HEHS-99-46	16. Improve the effectiveness of civil monetary penalties: The Administrator should continue to take those steps necessary to shorten the delay in adjudicating appeals, including monitoring progress made in reducing the backlog of appeals.	As requested by HHS, Congress approved increased funding and staffing levels for the Departmental Appeals Board in fiscal years 1999 and 2000.	●
	17. Strengthen the use and effect of termination:	CMS conducted a study and concluded that it was not practical to establish rules to address this problem.	◑
	• Continue Medicare and Medicaid payments beyond the termination date only if the home and state Medicaid agency are making reasonable efforts to transfer residents to other homes or alternative modes of care.		
	• Ensure that reasonable assurance periods associated with reinstating terminated homes are of sufficient duration to effectively demonstrate that the reason for termination has been resolved and will not recur.	CMS added examples to the reasonable assurance guidance in 2000, but declined to lengthen the reasonable assurance period.	
	• Strengthen the use and effect of termination: Revise existing policies so that the pretermination	In 2000, CMS revised its guidance so that pretermination history of a home is considered in taking subsequent enforcement actions.	

Table 2. (Continued)

GAO report number	GAO recommendation	CMS initiative	Implementation status
	history of a home is considered in taking a subsequent enforcement action.		
	18. Improve the referral process: The Administrator should revise CMS guidance so that states refer homes to CMS for possible sanction (such as civil monetary penalties) if they have been cited for a deficiency that contributed to a resident's death.	In 2000, CMS revised its guidance to require states to refer homes for possible sanction if they had been cited for a deficiency that contributed to a resident's death.	●
GAO-07-241	19. Reassess and revise the immediate sanctions policy to ensure that it accomplishes the following:	CMS acknowledged that the complexity of its immediate sanctions policy may be an inherent limitation and indicated that it intends to either strengthen the policy or replace it with a policy that achieves similar goals through alternative methods.	○
	• Reduce the lag time between citation of a double G and the implementation of a sanction.	CMS agreed to reduce the lag time between citation and implementation of a double G immediate sanction by limiting the prospective effective date for DPNAs to no more than 30 to 60 days.	
	• Prevent nursing homes that repeatedly harm residents or place them in immediate jeopardy from escaping sanctions.	CMS indicated it will remove the limitation in the double G policy on applying an additional sanction simply because a nursing home has not completed corrections to a deficiency that gave rise to a previous sanction.	
	• Hold states accountable for reporting in federal data systems serious deficiencies identified during complaint investigations so that all complaint findings are considered in determining when immediate sanctions are warranted.	CMS agreed to collect additional information on complaints for which data are not reported in federal data systems.	
	20. Strengthen the deterrent effect of available sanctions and ensure that sanctions are used to their fullest potential:		○
	• Ensure the consistency of CMPs by issuing guidance, such as the standardized CMP grid piloted during 2006.	CMS agreed to issue a CMP analytic tool, or grid, and to provide states with further guidance on discretionary DPNAs and terminations.	
	• Increase use of discretionary DPNAs to help ensure the speedier implementation of appropriate sanctions.	CMS indicated it will issue further guidance for states on factors to be considered in determining whether a discretionary DPNA is imposed or a termination date is set earlier than the time periods required by law	
	• Strengthen the criteria for terminating homes with a history of serious, repeated noncompliance by	CMS stated it will work with states, consumer organizations, stakeholders, and others to design	

Table 2. (Continued)

GAO report number	GAO recommendation	CMS initiative	Implementation status
	limiting the extension of termination dates, increasing the use of discretionary terminations, and exploring alternative thresholds for termination, such as the cumulative duration of noncompliance.	proposals for a better combination of enforcement actions for homes with repeated quality-of-care deficiencies.	
	21. Develop an administrative process under which CMPs would be paid—or Medicare and Medicaid payments in equivalent amounts would be withheld—prior to exhaustion of appeals and seek legislation for the implementation of this process, as appropriate.	CMS agreed to seek legislative authority to collect CMPs prior to the exhaustion of appeals.	○
	22. Further expand the Special Focus Facility program with enhanced enforcement requirements to include all homes that meet a threshold to qualify as poorly performing homes.	CMS agreed with the concept of expanding the Special Focus Facility program to include all homes that meet a threshold qualifying them as poorly performing homes, but said it lacks the resources needed for this expansion. CMS also identified other initiatives it will implement to improve the program.	○
	23. Improve the effectiveness of the new enforcement data system:		○
	• Develop the enforcement-related data systems' abilities to interface with each other in order to improve the tracking and monitoring of enforcement.	CMS agreed to study the feasibility of linking the separate data systems used for enforcement; however, it indicated that available resources may limit further action.	
	• Expedite the development of national enforcement reports and a concrete plan for using the reports.	CMS agreed to study the feasibility of developing national standard enforcement reports, but stated that further action on these reports may be limited by resource availability.	
	• Develop and institute a system of quality checks to ensure the accuracy and integrity of AEM data.	CMS agreed to develop and implement a system of quality checks to ensure the accuracy of its data systems, including AEM.	
	24. Expand CMS's Nursing Home Compare Web site to include implemented sanctions and homes subjected to immediate sanctions.	CMS proposed reporting implemented sanctions only for poorly performing homes that meet an undefined threshold—this is not fully responsive to our recommendation.	◑
Oversight			
GAO/HEHS-99-46	25. Develop better management information systems. The Administrator should enhance OSCAR or develop some other information system that can be used by both by the states and CMS to integrate the results of complaint investigations, track the status and history of deficiencies, and monitor enforcement actions.	CMS has implemented new national enforcement and complaint tracking systems but has delayed its replacement of the OSCAR data system until 2009 as a result of funding cuts and CMS focus on other initiatives.	○

Table 2. (Continued)

GAO report number	GAO recommendation	CMS initiative	Implementation status
GAO/HEHS-99-80	26. Require that the substantiated results of complaint investigations be included in federal data systems or be accessible by federal officials.	In January 2004, CMS's new ASPEN Complaint Tracking system was implemented nationwide.	●
GAO/HEHS-00-6	27. Improve the scope and rigor of CMS's oversight process:		●
	• Increase the proportion of federal monitoring surveys conducted as comparative surveys to ensure that a sufficient number are completed in each state to assess whether the state appropriately identifies serious deficiencies.	CMS has significantly increased the number of quality-of-care comparative surveys. In fiscal year 2006, however, the agency will no longer contract for additional quality-of-care comparative surveys because of funding constraints.	
	• Ensure that comparative surveys are initiated closer to the time the state agency completes the home's annual standard survey.	To better ensure that conditions in a nursing home have not changed since the state survey, CMS regional offices reduced the average time between the state survey and the initiation of a federal comparative survey from 33 days in 1999 to 26 days by 2004.	
	• Require regions to provide more timely written feedback to the states after the completion of federal monitoring surveys.	CMS instructed the regions to report the results of federal monitoring surveys to states on a monthly basis.	
	• Improve the data system for observational surveys so that it is an effective management tool for CMS to properly assess the findings of observational surveys.	CMS developed a separate database accessible to all regional offices that includes the results of observational surveys. Beginning in fiscal year 2002, CMS added data on the results of comparative surveys.	
	28. Improve the consistency in how CMS holds state survey agencies accountable by standardizing procedures for selecting state surveys and conducting federal monitoring surveys:		◑
	• Ensure that the regions target surveys for review that will provide a comprehensive assessment of state surveyor performance.	CMS did not implement our recommendation to select individual state surveys for federal review in a manner that ensures its regional offices observe as many state surveyors as possible.	
	• Require federal surveyors to include as many of the same residents as possible in their comparative survey sample as the state included in its sample (where CMS surveyors have determined that the state sample selection process was appropriate).	In October 2002, CMS instructed federal surveyors to select at least half of those residents selected by the state surveyors for their resident sample.	
	29. Further explore the feasibility of appropriate alternative remedies or sanctions for those states that prove unable or unwilling to meet CMS's performance standards.	In December 1999, CMS adopted new state sanctions. In fiscal year 2005, CMS began to tie survey agency funding increases to the	●

Table 2. (Continued)

GAO report number	GAO recommendation	CMS initiative	Implementation status
		timely conduct of standard surveys, a step that we believe offers a strong incentive for improved compliance.	
GAO/HEHS-02-279	30. Review the adequacy of current state efforts to ensure the accuracy of minimum data set (MDS) data, and provide, where necessary, additional guidance, training, and technical assistance.	CMS disagreed with and did not implement this recommendation.	⊗
	31. Monitor the adequacy of state MDS accuracy activities on an ongoing basis, such as through the use of the established federal comparative survey process.	CMS disagreed with and did not implement this recommendation.	⊗
	32. Provide guidance to state agencies and nursing homes that sufficient evidentiary documentation to support the full MDS assessment be included in residents' medical records.	CMS disagreed with and did not implement this recommendation.	⊗
GAO-03-187	33. Delay the implementation of nationwide reporting of quality indicators until there is greater assurance that the quality indicators are appropriate for public reporting—including the validity of the indicators selected and the use of an appropriate risk-adjustment methodology— based on input from the National Quality Forum and other experts and, if necessary, additional analysis and testing.	CMS disagreed with and did not implement this recommendation.	⊗
	34. Delay the implementation of nationwide reporting of quality indicators until a more thorough evaluation of the pilot is completed to help improve the initiative's effectiveness, including an assessment of the presentation of information on the Web site and the resources needed to assist consumers' use of the information.	CMS disagreed with and did not implement this recommendation.	⊗
GAO-03-561	35. Further refine annual state performance reviews so that they (1) consistently distinguish between systemic problems and less serious issues regarding state performance, (2) analyze trends in the proportion of homes that harm residents, (3) assess state compliance with the immediate sanctions policy for homes with a pattern of harming residents, and (4) analyze the predictability of state surveys.	CMS did not implement this recommendation because it believes that the state performance standards take into account statutory and nonstatutory performance standards.	⊗
GAO-04-660	36. Ensure that CMS regional offices fully comply with the statutory requirement to conduct annual federal monitoring surveys by including an assessment of the fire safety	CMS's evaluation of state surveyors' performance now routinely includes fire safety as part of the statutory requirement to annually conduct federal	●

Table 2. (Continued)

GAO report number	GAO recommendation	CMS initiative	Implementation status
	component of states' standard surveys, with an emphasis on unsprinklered homes.	monitoring surveys in at least 5 percent of surveyed nursing homes in each state.	
	37. Ensure that data on sprinkler coverage in nursing homes are consistently obtained and reflected in the CMS database.	CMS now obtains the sprinkler status of over 99 percent of nursing homes during routine surveys and inputs this information into OSCAR.	●
	38. Until sprinkler coverage data are routinely available in CMS's database, work with state survey agencies to identify the extent to which each nursing home is sprinklered or not sprinklered.	See CMS action in response to recommendation for ensuring that data on sprinkler coverage in nursing homes are consistently obtained (recommendation #37 above).	●
	39. On an expedited basis, review all waivers and Fire Safety Evaluation System (FSES) assessments for homes that are not fully sprinklered to determine their appropriateness.[b]	CMS has completed reviews of all waiver requests and FSES assessments and noted that the number of homes using FSES dropped significantly as a result of the review.	●
	40. Make information on fire safety deficiencies available to the public via the Nursing Home Compare Web site, including information on whether a home has automatic sprinklers.	This information was made available on the Nursing Home Compare Web site as of October 2006.	●
	41. Work with the National Fire Protection Association to strengthen fire safety standards for unsprinklered nursing homes, such as requiring smoke detectors in resident rooms, exploring the feasibility of requiring sprinklers in all nursing homes, and developing a strategy for financing such requirements.	CMS issued regulations effective May 24, 2005, requiring nursing facilities to install smoke detectors in resident rooms and public areas if they do not have a sprinkler system installed throughout the facility or a hard-wired smoke detection system in those areas. Facilities were given 1 year, until May 24, 2006, to comply with this requirement. In addition, the National Fire Protection Association approved a revision to the 2006 Life Safety Code which requires the installation of automatic sprinkler systems in all existing facilities.	●
	42. Ensure that thorough investigations are conducted following multiple-death nursing home fires so that fire safety standards can be reevaluated and modified where appropriate.	CMS developed and issued a standardized procedure to ensure that both state survey agencies and its own staff take appropriate action to investigate fires that result in serious injury or death.	●

(●) Fully implemented our recommendation

(◑) Implemented only part of our recommendation and no further steps are planned

(○) Taking steps to implement our recommendation

(⊗) Did not implement our recommendation

Source: GAO analysis of CMS's responses to our recommendations.

[a] In 1999, CMS had required the use of an investigative protocol on abuse prohibition during every standard survey. The protocol's objective is to determine if the facility has developed and operationalized policies and procedures that prohibit abuse, neglect, involuntary seclusion, and misappropriation of resident property.

[b] As an alternative to correcting or receiving a waiver for deficiencies identified on a standard survey, a home may undergo an assessment using the Fire Safety Evaluation System. The system provides a means for nursing homes to meet the fire safety objectives of CMS's standards without necessarily being in full compliance with every standard.

Table 2 summarizes our recommendations from 11 reports on nursing home quality and safety, issued from July 1998 through March 2007; CMS's actions to address weaknesses we identified; and the implementation status of CMS's initiatives as of April 2007. The recommendations are grouped into four categories—surveys, complaints, enforcement, and oversight. If a report contained recommendations related to more than one category, the report appears more than once in the table. For each report, the first two numbers identify the fiscal year in which the report was issued. For example, HEHS-98-202 was released in 1998. The Related GAO Products section at the end of this statement contains the full citation for each report. Of our 42 recommendations, CMS has fully implemented 18, implemented only parts of 7, is taking steps to implement 10, and declined to implement 7.

APPENDIX II: PERCENTAGE OF NURSING HOMES CITED FOR ACTUAL HARM OR IMMEDIATE JEOPARDY DURING STANDARD SURVEYS

In order to identify trends in the percentage of nursing homes cited with actual harm or immediate jeopardy deficiencies, we analyzed data from CMS's OSCAR database for fiscal years 2000 through 2006 (see table 3). Because surveys are conducted at least every 15 months (with a required 12-month statewide average), it is possible that a home was surveyed twice in any time period. To avoid double counting of homes, we included only homes' most recent survey from each period.

Table 3. Percentage of Nursing Homes Cited for Actual Harm or Immediate Jeopardy, by State, Fiscal Years 2000-2006

	Fiscal year							
State	**Number of homes 2006**	**2000**	**2001**	**2002**	**2003**	**2004**	**2005**	**2006**
Alabama	231	35.5	23.0	12.7	18.1	15.6	23.1	24.2
Alaska	15	28.6	26.7	26.7	0.0	0.0	0.0	26.7
Arizona	135	24.2	12.6	7.3	6.6	9.4	9.9	24.8
Arkansas	245	38.1	27.7	22.3	24.7	19.5	15.9	14.5
California	1,304	24.1	10.9	5.1	3.7	6.1	8.0	14.1
Colorado	215	20.4	26.4	32.7	20.9	25.9	40.4	44.8
Connecticut	245	41.9	51.6	45.8	43.1	54.4	44.2	50.8
Delaware	44	47.5	14.6	10.8	5.3	15.0	35.7	36.8
District of Columbia	20	17.7	28.6	30.0	41.2	40.0	30.0	25.0
Florida	688	22.8	20.2	14.9	10.2	7.8	4.2	9.1
Georgia	371	19.5	21.0	23.7	24.6	16.6	18.0	15.9
Hawaii	48	23.8	14.3	21.2	12.1	22.9	2.8	2.1
Idaho	80	51.4	29.7	39.2	31.9	27.3	38.4	47.8
Illinois	816	28.4	19.2	15.3	18.3	15.1	15.7	21.7
Indiana	526	45.0	29.4	23.2	19.7	24.1	28.3	33.4
Iowa	466	14.7	12.0	8.0	9.1	11.8	11.2	11.7

Table 3. (Continued)

Kansas	361	37.9	30.7	32.9	26.5	30.3	34.9	38.3
Kentucky	298	26.8	29.1	23.2	26.1	14.6	7.7	11.4
Louisiana	307	21.8	29.9	21.7	16.2	12.0	15.4	15.8
Maine	114	11.1	13.9	6.6	11.1	12.8	7.0	9.8
Maryland	235	22.4	16.5	26.1	15.4	17.8	7.6	7.6
Massachusetts	456	29.1	24.4	24.6	25.9	16.7	22.6	20.9
Michigan	429	42.8	24.5	29.7	26.9	22.9	22.9	29.7
Minnesota	404	30.4	17.3	22.3	18.3	14.3	14.4	18.8
Mississippi	207	33.0	19.8	18.7	16.0	18.9	18.1	9.4
Missouri	526	19.8	13.0	15.6	12.5	11.7	15.4	15.6
Montana	97	33.3	29.7	12.0	20.0	18.0	17.9	16.7
Nebraska	229	19.2	21.1	20.1	14.8	15.3	14.4	25.7
Nevada	47	34.8	14.6	11.9	9.1	17.5	19.6	21.3
New Hampshire	83	37.8	31.1	29.4	24.1	25.6	26.3	22.9
New Jersey	363	25.5	27.8	18.8	10.5	13.5	18.2	15.5
New Mexico	75	23.7	16.9	14.9	21.3	24.3	29.4	25.0
New York	658	33.8	37.1	34.2	15.2	11.0	14.0	18.5
North Carolina	424	43.6	35.8	25.6	29.0	21.1	18.5	17.2
				Fiscal year				
State	**Number of homes 2006**	**2000**	**2001**	**2002**	**2003**	**2004**	**2005**	**2006**
North Dakota	83	25.9	28.7	17.9	12.4	13.6	17.7	21.7
Ohio	980	26.6	27.3	25.4	19.1	11.4	13.8	14.6
Oklahoma	359	19.3	21.3	22.0	26.3	13.9	23.2	20.1
Oregon	142	45.5	32.6	23.7	20.3	15.9	19.8	18.6
Pennsylvania	724	30.3	19.2	13.5	17.2	19.5	15.2	13.6
Rhode Island	90	14.3	12.9	5.6	6.7	9.3	9.5	4.5
South Carolina	178	26.4	17.2	19.8	29.6	32.7	24.8	17.1
South Dakota	111	27.1	26.7	26.8	32.1	21.6	12.8	21.7
Tennessee	332	28.2	20.2	20.7	21.8	22.9	17.3	12.5
Texas	1,175	29.7	30.5	22.4	18.0	12.0	16.2	18.3
Utah	93	19.5	14.1	25.6	19.0	11.1	8.4	17.9
Vermont	41	22.5	18.2	15.0	10.0	19.5	23.7	13.5
Virginia	281	19.2	14.3	11.6	13.7	10.2	15.5	15.8
Washington	247	46.9	38.3	37.0	30.9	28.1	27.2	24.1
West Virginia	132	12.1	17.7	20.4	12.7	9.8	15.0	9.7
Wisconsin	403	15.8	15.6	11.2	10.9	13.1	18.2	23.0
Wyoming	39	52.8	32.4	25.0	22.9	17.1	11.8	16.2
Nation	**16,172**	**28.4**	**23.3**	**20.2**	**17.8**	**15.7**	**16.8**	**18.9**

Source: GAO analysis of OSCAR and PDQ data.

Related GAO Products

Nursing Homes: Efforts to Strengthen Federal Enforcement Have Not Deterred Some Homes from Repeatedly Harming Residents. GAO-07-241. Washington, D.C.: March 26, 2007.

Nursing Homes: Despite Increased Oversight, Challenges Remain in Ensuring High-Quality Care and Resident Safety. GAO-06-117. Washington, D.C.: December 28, 2005.

Nursing Home Deaths: Arkansas Coroner Referrals Confirm Weaknesses in State and Federal Oversight of Quality of Care. GAO-05-78. Washington, D.C.: November 12, 2004.

Nursing Home Fire Safety: Recent Fires Highlight Weaknesses in Federal Standards and Oversight. GAO-04-660. Washington D.C.: July 16, 2004.
Nursing Home Quality: Prevalence of Serious Problems, While Declining, Reinforces Importance of Enhanced Oversight. GAO-03-561. Washington, D.C.: July 15, 2003.
Nursing Homes: Public Reporting of Quality Indicators Has Merit, but National Implementation Is Premature. GAO-03-187. Washington, D.C.: October 31, 2002.
Nursing Homes: Quality of Care More Related to Staffing than Spending. GAO-02-431R. Washington, D.C.: June 13, 2002.
Nursing Homes: More Can Be Done to Protect Residents from Abuse. GAO-02-312. Washington, D.C.: March 1, 2002.
Nursing Homes: Federal Efforts to Monitor Resident Assessment Data Should Complement State Activities. GAO-02-279. Washington, D.C.: February 15, 2002.
Nursing Homes: Sustained Efforts Are Essential to Realize Potential of the Quality Initiatives. GAO/HEHS-00-197. Washington, D.C.: September 28, 2000.
Nursing Home Care: Enhanced HCFA Oversight of State Programs Would Better Ensure Quality. GAO/HEHS-00-6. Washington, D.C.: November 4, 1999.
Nursing Home Oversight: Industry Examples Do Not Demonstrate That Regulatory Actions Were Unreasonable. GAO/HEHS-99-154R. Washington, D.C.: August 13, 1999.
Nursing Homes: Proposal to Enhance Oversight of Poorly Performing Homes Has Merit. GAO/HEHS-99-157. Washington, D.C.: June 30, 1999.
Nursing Homes: Complaint Investigation Processes Often Inadequate to Protect Residents. GAO/HEHS-99-80. Washington, D.C.: March 22, 1999.
Nursing Homes: Additional Steps Needed to Strengthen Enforcement of Federal Quality Standards. GAO/HEHS-99-46. Washington, D.C.: March 18, 1999.
California Nursing Homes: Care Problems Persist Despite Federal and State Oversight. GAO/HEHS-98-202. Washington, D.C.: July 27, 1998.

End Notes

[1] See Institute of Medicine, National Academy of Sciences, *Improving the Quality of Care in Nursing Homes* (Washington, D.C.: March 1986).

[2] GAO, *Medicare and Medicaid: Stronger Enforcement of Nursing Home Requirements Needed*, GAO/HRD-87-113 (Washington, D.C.: July 22, 1987).

[3] Prior to July 2001, CMS was known as the Health Care Financing Administration. Throughout this testimony, we refer to the agency as CMS, even when describing initiatives taken prior to its name change. Medicare is the federal health care program for elderly and disabled people. Medicare may cover up to 100 days of skilled nursing home care following a hospital stay. Medicaid is the joint federal-state health care financing program for certain categories of low-income individuals. Medicaid also pays for long-term care services, including nursing home care.

[4] In this chapter, we use the term states to include the 50 states and the District of Columbia.

[5] Related GAO products are included at the end of this statement. See appendix I for recommendations GAO has made, related CMS initiatives, and the implementation status of these initiatives.

[6] OBRA '87 included other requirements pertaining to nursing homes, such as staffing, services, and specific rights of residents, including privacy, restricted use of physical or chemical restraints, and voicing of grievances, but GAO has not examined these issues.

[7] CMS generally interprets these requirements to permit a statewide average interval of 12.9 months and a maximum interval of 15.9 months for each home. In addition to nursing homes, CMS and state survey agencies are responsible for oversight of other Medicare and Medicaid providers such as home health agencies, intermediate care facilities for the mentally retarded, accredited and nonaccredited hospitals, end-stage renal dialysis facilities, ambulatory surgical centers, rural health clinics, outpatient physical therapy

centers, hospices, portable x-ray suppliers, comprehensive outpatient rehabilitation facilities, and Community Mental Health Centers.

[8] CMS contracts with state survey agencies to conduct surveys and complaint investigations.

[9] CMS requires nursing homes to meet applicable provisions of the fire safety standards developed by the National Fire Protection Association (NFPA), of which CMS is a member. NFPA is a nonprofit membership organization that develops and advocates scientifically based consensus standards on fire, building, and electrical safety.

[10] Ensuring that documented deficiencies are corrected is a shared federal-state responsibility. States are responsible for enforcing standards in homes with Medicaid-only certification—about 14 percent of homes. They may use the federal sanctions or rely on their own state licensure authority and nursing home sanctions.

[11] As of December 2004, Alaska is not required to select Special Focus Facilities, because there were fewer than 21 nursing homes in the state at that time.

[12] If efforts to collect the CMP directly from the home fail, Medicare and Medicaid payments are withheld.

[13] Homes also can choose to close voluntarily, but we do not consider voluntary closure to be a sanction. When a home is terminated, it loses any income from Medicare and Medicaid, which accounted for about 40 percent of nursing home payments in 2004. Residents who receive support through Medicare or Medicaid must be moved to other facilities. However, a terminated home generally can apply for reinstatement if it corrects its deficiencies.

[14] GAO, *Nursing Homes: Despite Increased Oversight, Challenges Remain in Ensuring High-Quality Care and Resident Safety*, GAO-06-117 (Washington, D.C.: Dec. 28, 2005).

[15] For example, a deficiency noted in a federal survey could involve a resident who was not in the nursing home at the time of the state survey.

[16] GAO-06-117. CMS requires its federal surveyors to specifically identify which deficiencies state surveyors missed during the state survey.

[17] These declines in serious deficiencies were 14.3 percentage points for Texas, 15.4 percentage points for Florida, 17.4 percentage points for Ohio, 22.8 percentage points for California, and 23.0 percentage points for New York.

[18] GAO, *Nursing Homes: Efforts to Strengthen Federal Enforcement Have Not Deterred Some Homes from Repeatedly Harming Residents*, GAO-07-241 (Washington, D.C.: Mar. 26, 2007).

[19] GAO-07-241. In this chapter, we analyzed federal sanctions from fiscal year 2000 through 2005 against 63 nursing homes with a history of harming residents and whose prior compliance and enforcement histories formed the basis for the conclusions in our March 1999 report. The homes were located in California, Michigan, Pennsylvania, and Texas.

[20] In 2003, we reported that we found over 700 cases that should have been referred for immediate sanctions but were not, from January 2000 through March 2002. See GAO, *Nursing Home Quality: Prevalence of Serious Problems, While Declining, Reinforces Importance of Enhanced Oversight*, GAO-03-561 (Washington, D.C.: July 15, 2003).

[21] CMPs and DPNAs accounted for 80 percent of federal sanctions from fiscal year 2000 through 2005. The majority of federal sanctions implemented during this time period— about 54 percent—were CMPs. During this time period, DPNAs and terminations accounted for about 26 percent and less than 1 percent of federal sanctions, respectively.

[22] See HHS, Office of Inspector General, *Nursing Home Enforcement: The Use of Civil Money Penalties*, OEI-06-02-00720 (April 2005).

[23] Use of the CMP grid would be optional to provide states flexibility to tailor sanctions to specific circumstances.

[24] We recently recommended that the Administrator of CMS undertake a number of steps to strengthen enforcement capabilities. CMS generally concurred with our recommendations, although it pointed out some resource constraints to implementing certain ones. See GAO-07-241.

[25] Annual state performance reviews were established in fiscal year 2001 and fully implemented in fiscal year 2002.

[26] GAO-06-117.

[27] Pilot programs have been phased in from fall 2005 through September 2007 in seven states—Alaska, Idaho, Illinois, Michigan, Nevada, New Mexico, and Wisconsin. An independent evaluation is expected in spring 2008.

[28] As of fiscal year 2006, there were about 16,000 nursing homes which would require over 800 federal monitoring surveys. Since 1992 when all federal monitoring surveys were comparative, CMS has begun to rely more heavily on observational surveys, which require a smaller number of federal surveyors. In fiscal year 2006, roughly 77 percent of federal monitoring surveys were observational.

[29] GAO, *Nursing Home Fire Safety: Recent Fires Highlight Weaknesses in Federal Standards and Oversight*, GAO-04-660 (Washington D.C.: July 16, 2004).

[30] 71 Fed. Reg. 55326 (Sept. 22, 2006) (codified in pertinent part at 42 C.F.R. §483. 70). CMS began surveying nursing homes' compliance with the new requirement in May 2006.

[31] 71 Fed. Reg. 62957 (Oct. 27, 2006) (to be codified at 42 C.F.R. §483.70).

[32] http://www.medicare.gov/NHCompare/home.asp.

[33]GAO, *Nursing Homes: Federal Efforts to Monitor Resident Assessment Data Should Complement State Activities*, GAO-02-279 (Washington, D.C.: Feb. 15, 2002).

In: Nursing Homes Quality and Care Issues
Editor: Carlos E. Melendez
ISBN: 978-1-61668-855-4

Chapter 2

Nursing Homes: Addressing the Factors Underlying Understatement of Serious Care Problems Requires Sustained CMS and State Commitment*

Government Accountability Office

Why GAO Did This Study

Under contract with the CMS, states conduct surveys at nursing homes to help ensure compliance with federal quality standards. Over the past decade, GAO has reported on inconsistencies in states' assessment of nursing homes' quality of care, including understatement—that is, when state surveys fail to cite serious deficiencies or cite them at too low a level. In 2008, GAO reported that 9 states had high and 10 had low understatement based on CMS data for fiscal years 2002 through 2007. This chapter examines the effect on nursing home deficiency understatement of CMS's survey process, workforce shortages and training, supervisory reviews of surveys, and state agency practices. GAO primarily collected data through two Web-based questionnaires sent to all eligible nursing home surveyors and state agency directors, achieving 61 and 98 percent response rates, respectively.

What GAO Recommends

GAO is making seven recommendations to the CMS Administrator to address state and surveyor issues about CMS's survey methodology and guidance, workforce shortages and insufficient training, inconsistencies in the focus and frequency of the supervisory review of deficiencies, and external pressure from the nursing home industry. CMS concurred with five

* This is an edited, reformatted and augmented version of a U. S. Government Accountability Office publication dated November 2009.

of GAO's seven recommendations and indicated it would explore alternate solutions to the remaining two recommendations.

WHAT GAO FOUND

A substantial percentage of both state surveyors and directors identified general weaknesses in the nursing home survey process, that is, the survey methodology and guidance on identifying deficiencies. On the questionnaires, 46 percent of surveyors and 36 percent of directors reported that weaknesses in the traditional survey methodology, such as too many survey tasks, contributed to understatement. Limited experience with a new data-driven survey methodology indicated possible improvements in consistency; however, an independent evaluation led CMS to conclude that other tools, such as survey guidance clarification and surveyor training and supervision, would help improve survey accuracy.

According to questionnaire responses, workforce shortages and greater use of surveyors with less than 2 years' experience sometimes contributed to understatement. Nearly three-quarters of directors reported that they always or frequently experienced a workforce shortage, while nearly two-thirds reported that surveyor inexperience always, frequently, or sometimes led to understatement. Substantial percentages of directors and surveyors indicated that inadequate training may compromise survey accuracy and lead to understatement. According to about 29 percent of surveyors in 9 high understatement states compared to 16 percent of surveyors in 10 low understatement states, initial surveyor training was not sufficient to cite appropriate scope and severity—a skill critical in preventing understatement. Furthermore, over half of directors identified the need for ongoing training for experienced surveyors on both this skill and on documenting deficiencies, a critical skill to substantiate citations.

CMS provides little guidance to states on supervisory review processes. In general, directors reported on our questionnaire that supervisory reviews occurred more often on surveys with higher-level rather than on those with lower-level deficiencies, which were the most frequently understated. Surveyors who reported that survey teams had too many new surveyors also reported frequent changes to or removal of deficiencies, indicating heavier reliance on supervisory reviews by states with inexperienced surveyors.

Surveyors and directors in a few states informed us that, in isolated cases, state agency practices or external pressure from stakeholders, such as the nursing home industry, may have led to understatement. Forty percent of surveyors in five states and four directors reported that their state had at least one practice not to cite certain deficiencies. Additionally, over 40 percent of surveyors in four states reported that their states' informal dispute resolution processes favored concerns of nursing home operators over resident welfare. Furthermore, directors from seven states reported that pressure from the industry or legislators may have compromised the nursing home survey process, and two directors reported that CMS's support is needed to deal with such pressure. If surveyors perceive that certain deficiencies may not be consistently upheld or enforced, they may choose not to cite them.

ABBREVIATIONS

AHFSA	Association of Health Facility Survey Agencies
CMS	Centers for Medicare & Medicaid Services
HHS	Department of Health & Human Services
IDR	Informal Dispute Resolution
OSCAR	On-Line Survey, Certification, and Reporting system
RN	registered nurse
SMQT	Surveyor Minimum Qualifications Test
SOM	State Operations Manual
QIS	Quality Indicator Survey

November 24, 2009

The Honorable Herb Kohl
Chairman
Special Committee on Aging
United States Senate

The Honorable Charles E. Grassley
Ranking Member
Committee on Finance
United States Senate

Federal and state governments share responsibility for ensuring that nursing homes provide quality care in a safe environment for the nation's 1.5 million residents dependent on such care. The federal government is responsible for setting quality requirements that nursing homes must meet to participate in the Medicare and Medicaid programs.[1] The Centers for Medicare & Medicaid Services (CMS), within the Department of Health & Human Services (HHS), contracts with state survey agencies to conduct periodic inspections, known as surveys, and complaint investigations, both of which assess whether homes meet federal standards.[2] State survey agencies are required to follow federal regulations for surveying facilities; however, several survey activities and policies are left largely to the discretion of state survey agencies, including hiring and retaining a surveyor workforce, training surveyors, reviewing deficiency citations, and managing regulatory interactions with the industry and public.

In response to congressional requests over the last decade, we have reported significant weaknesses in federal and state activities designed to detect and correct quality and safety problems in nursing homes and the persistence of serious deficiencies, which are those deficiencies that harm residents or place them at risk of death or serious injury.[3] In the course of our work, we regularly found significant variation across states in their citations of serious deficiencies—indicating inconsistencies in states' assessment of quality of care. We also found evidence of substantial understatement—that is, state inspections that failed to cite serious deficiencies or that cited deficiencies at too low a level.

In this chapter, we complete our response to your request to examine the understatement of serious deficiencies in nursing homes by state surveyors nationwide and the factors that contribute to understatement. Our first report, issued in May 2008, identified the extent of nursing home understatement nationwide.[4] It found that 15 percent of federal nursing home surveys nationwide and 25 percent of these surveys in nine states identified state surveys that failed to cite serious deficiencies. This chapter examines how the following factors affect the understatement of nursing home deficiencies: (1) the CMS survey process, (2) workforce shortages and training, (3) supervisory reviews, and (4) state agency practices.

To do this work, we analyzed data collected from two GAO-administered Web-based questionnaires, one to nursing home surveyors and the other to state agency directors; analyzed federal and state nursing home survey results; interviewed CMS officials from the Survey and Certification Group and selected Regional Offices; reviewed federal regulations and guidance, and our prior work; and conducted follow-up interviews with state agency directors, as needed, to clarify and better understand their unique state circumstances.[5]

Our prior work documented the prevalence of understatement nationwide and described several factors that may contribute to survey inconsistency and the understatement of deficiencies by state survey teams: (1) weaknesses in CMS's survey methodology, including poor documentation of deficiencies,[6] (2) confusion among surveyors about the definition of actual harm,[7] (3) predictability of surveys, which allows homes to conceal problems if they so desire,[8] (4) inadequate quality assurance processes at the state level to help detect understatement in the scope and severity of deficiencies,[9] and (5) inexperienced state surveyors as a result of retention problems.[10] We relied on this information and feedback from pretests with six surveyors from a local state and five current or former state agency directors to develop our questionnaires on the nursing home survey process and factors that contribute to the understatement of deficiencies.

Our Web-based questionnaires of nursing home surveyors and state agency directors achieved response rates of 61 percent and 98 percent, respectively. The first questionnaire collected responses from 2,340 of the total 3,819 eligible nursing home surveyors in 49 states and the District of Columbia.[11] The resulting sample of surveyors who responded to our questionnaire between May and July 2008 was representative of surveyors nationally, with the exception of Pennsylvania.[12] Fifty state agency directors responded to the second questionnaire from September to November 2008.[13] Many questions on our questionnaires asked respondents to identify the frequency that an event occurred using the following scale—always, frequently, sometimes, infrequently, or never; however, for reporting purposes, we grouped responses into three categories—always/frequently, sometimes, and infrequently/never. In addition, our questionnaire to state agency directors asked them to rank the degree to which several factors, derived from our previous work, contributed to understatement.[14] Summary results from the GAO questionnaires are available as an e-supplement to this chapter. See *Nursing Homes: Responses from Two Web-Based Questionnaires to Nursing Home Surveyors and State Agency Directors* (GAO-10-74SP), an e-supplement to GAO-10-70.

We analyzed the data collected from these questionnaires as stand-alone datasets and in relationship to state performance on federal comparative and observational surveys as captured in the federal monitoring survey database, which we reported on in 2008.[15] In addition, to inform our understanding of the extent to which each factor contributed to understatement, we examined relationships among the responses to both questionnaires and the results of the federal comparative and observational surveys for fiscal years 2002 through 2007. We used the results of the federal comparative surveys for these years to identify states with high and low percentages of serious missed deficiencies. We report results for tests of association and differences between group averages.

We also interviewed directors and other state agency officials in eight states to better understand unusual or interesting circumstances related to surveyor workforce and training, supervisory review, or state policies and practices. We selected these eight state agencies based on our analysis of questionnaire responses from the state agency directors and nursing home surveyors.

To compare average facility citations on state survey records with the average citations on federal survey records, we collected information from the On-Line Survey, Certification, and Reporting (OSCAR) system for those facilities where federal teams assessed state surveyor performance for fiscal years 2002 through 2007.[16] Except where otherwise noted, we used data from fiscal year 2007 because they were the most recently available data at the time of our analysis (see appendix I for more on our scope and methodology).

We conducted this performance audit from April 2008 through November 2009 in accordance with generally accepted government auditing standards. Those standards require that we plan and perform the audit to obtain sufficient, appropriate evidence to provide a reasonable basis for our findings and conclusions based on our audit objectives. We believe that the evidence obtained provides a reasonable basis for our findings and conclusions based on our audit objectives.

BACKGROUND

Oversight of nursing homes is a shared federal-state responsibility. As part of this responsibility, CMS (1) sets federal quality standards, (2) establishes state responsibilities for ensuring federal quality standards are met, (3) issues guidance on determining compliance with these standards, and (4) performs oversight of state survey activities. It communicates these federal standards and state responsibilities in the State Operations Manual (SOM) and through special communications such as program memorandums and survey and certification letters. CMS provides less guidance on how states should manage the administration of their survey programs.

Table 1. Scope and Severity of Deficiencies Identified during Nursing Home Surveys

Severity	Scope		
	Isolated	Pattern	Widespread
Immediate jeopardy[a]	J	K	L
Actual harm	G	H	I
Potential for more than minimal harm	D	E	F
Potential for minimal harm[b]	A	B	C

Source: CMS.

[a] Actual or potential for death / serious injury.

[b] Nursing home is considered to be in "substantial compliance."

CMS uses staff in its 10 regional offices to oversee states' performance on surveys that ensure that facilities participating in Medicare and Medicaid provide high-quality care in a safe environment. Yet, the persistent understatement of serious nursing home deficiencies that we have reported and survey quality weaknesses that we and the HHS Office of Inspector General identified serve as indicators of weaknesses in the federal, state, or shared components of oversight.

Survey Process

Every nursing home receiving Medicare or Medicaid payment must undergo a standard state survey not less than once every 15 months, and the statewide average interval for these surveys must not exceed 12 months. During a standard survey, teams of state surveyors—generally consisting of registered nurses, social workers, dieticians, or other specialists—evaluate compliance with federal quality standards. The survey team determines whether the care and services provided meet the assessed needs of the residents and measure resident outcomes, such as the incidence of preventable pressure sores, weight loss, and accidents. In contrast to a standard survey, a complaint investigation generally focuses on a specific allegation regarding a resident's care or safety and provides an opportunity for state surveyors to intervene promptly if problems arise between standard surveys.

Surveyors assess facilities using federal nursing home quality standards that focus on the delivery of care, resident outcomes, and facility conditions. These standards total approximately 200 and are grouped into 15 categories, such as Quality of Life, Resident Assessment, Quality of Care, and Administration.[17] For example, there are 23 standards (known as F-tags) within the Quality of Care category ranging from the prevention of pressure sore development (F-314) to keeping the resident environment as free of accident hazards (F-323) as is possible.

Surveyors categorize deficient practices identified on standard surveys and complaint investigations—facilities' failures to meet federal standards—according to scope (i.e., the number of residents potentially or actually affected) and severity (i.e., the degree of relative harm involved)—using a scope and severity grid (see table 1). Homes with deficiencies at the A through C levels are considered to be in substantial compliance, while those with deficiencies at the D through L levels are considered out of compliance. Throughout this chapter, we refer to deficiencies at the actual harm and immediate jeopardy levels—G through L—as serious deficiencies. CMS guidance requires state survey teams to revisit a home to verify that serious deficiencies have actually been corrected.[18]

In addition, when serious deficiencies are identified, sanctions can be imposed to encourage facilities to correct the deficiencies and enforce federal quality standards. Sanctions include fines known as civil money penalties, denial of payment for new Medicare or Medicaid admissions, or termination from the Medicare and Medicaid programs. For example, facilities that receive at least one G through L level deficiency on successive standard surveys or complaint investigations must be referred for immediate sanctions. Facilities may appeal cited deficiencies and if the appeal is successful, the severity of the sanction could be reduced or the sanction could be rescinded. Facilities have several avenues of appeal, including informal dispute resolution (IDR) at the state survey agency level.[19] The

IDR gives providers one opportunity to informally refute cited deficiencies after any survey. While CMS requires that states have an IDR policy in place, it does not specify how IDR processes should be structured.

Survey Methodology

To conduct nursing home surveys, CMS has traditionally used a methodology that requires surveyors to select a sample of residents and (1) review data derived from the residents' assessments and medical records; (2) interview nursing home staff, residents, and family members; and (3) observe care provided to residents during the course of the survey. When conducting a survey, surveyors have discretion in: selecting a sample of residents to evaluate; allocating survey time and emphasis within a framework prescribed by CMS; investigating potentially deficient practices observed during the survey; and determining what evidence is needed to identify a deficient practice. CMS has developed detailed investigative protocols to assist state survey agencies in determining whether nursing homes are in compliance with federal quality standards. These protocols are intended to ensure the thoroughness and consistency of state surveys and complaint investigations.

In 1998, CMS awarded a contract to revise the survey methodology. The new Quality Indicator Survey (QIS) was developed to improve the consistency and efficiency of state surveys and provide a more reliable assessment of quality. The QIS uses an expanded sample of residents and structured interviews with residents and family members in a two-stage process. Surveyors are guided through the QIS process using customized software on tablet personal computers. In stage 1, a large resident sample is drawn and relevant data from on- and off-site sources is analyzed to develop a set of quality-of-care indicators, which will be compared to national benchmarks.[20] Stage 2 systematically investigates potential quality-of-care concerns identified in stage 1. Because of delays in implementing the QIS, we recommended in 2003 that CMS finalize the development, testing, and implementation of a more rigorous survey methodology, including investigative protocols that provide guidance to surveyors in documenting deficiencies at the appropriate scope and severity level.[21] CMS concluded a five-state demonstration process of the QIS in 2007 and is currently expanding the implementation of the QIS. As of 2008, only Connecticut had implemented the QIS statewide, and CMS projected that the QIS would not be fully implemented in every state until 2014.

State Administration

States are largely responsible for the administration of the survey program. State survey agencies administer and have discretion over many survey activities and policies, including hiring and retaining a surveyor workforce, training surveyors, conducting supervisory reviews of surveys, and other activities.

- *Hiring and Retaining a Surveyor Workforce:* State survey agencies hire the staff to conduct surveys of nursing homes and determine the salaries of these personnel according to the workforce practices and restrictions of the state. Salaries, particularly surveyor salaries, are the most significant cost component of state survey activities, which are supported through a combination of Medicare, Medicaid, and non-Medicaid state funds.[22] CMS has some requirements for the make-up of nursing home survey teams, including the involvement of at least one registered nurse (RN) in each nursing home survey. In February 2009, we reported that officials from the Association of Health Facility Survey Agencies (AHFSA) and other state officials told us they have had difficulty recruiting and retaining the survey workforce for several years. In our report, we recommended that CMS undertake a broad-based reexamination to ensure, among other aspects, an adequate survey workforce with sufficient compensation to attract and retain qualified staff.[23]

- *Training:* States are responsible for training new surveyors through participating in actual surveys under direct supervision. Within their first year of employment, surveyors must complete two CMS online training courses—the Basic Health Facility Surveyor Course and Principles of Documentation—and a week-long CMS-led Basic Long-Term Care Health Facility Surveyor Training Course; at the conclusion of the course surveyors must pass the Surveyor Minimum Qualifications Test (SMQT) to survey independently. In addition, state survey agencies are required to have their own programs for staff development that respond to the need for continuing development and education of both new and experienced employees. Such staff development programs must include training for surveyors on all regulatory requirements and the skills necessary to conduct surveys. To assist in continuing education, CMS develops a limited number of courses for ongoing training and provides other training materials.

- *Supervisory Reviews:* States may design a supervisory review process for deficiencies cited during surveys, although CMS does not require them to do so. In July 2003, we recommended that CMS require states to have a minimum quality-assurance process that includes a review of a sample of survey reports below the level of actual harm to assess the appropriateness of scope and severity levels cited and help reduce instances of understated quality-of-care problems.[24] CMS did not implement this recommendation.[25]

- *State Agency Practices and Policies:* State survey agencies' practices, including those on citing deficiencies and addressing pressure from the industry or others, are largely left to the discretion of state survey agencies. In the past, we reported that in one state, CMS officials had found surveyors were not citing all deficiencies.[26] If a state agency fails to cite all deficiencies associated with noncompliance, nursing home deficiencies are understated on the survey record. CMS can identify or monitor states for systematic noncitation practices through reviews of citation patterns, informal feedback from state surveyors, state performance reviews, and federal monitoring surveys (discussed below).[27] CMS also gives states latitude in defining their IDR process.

Federal Monitoring Surveys and Evidence of Understatement

Federal law requires federal surveyors to conduct federal monitoring surveys in at least 5 percent of state-surveyed Medicare and Medicaid nursing homes in each state each year. CMS indicates it meets the statutory requirement by conducting a mix of on-site reviews: comparative and observational surveys.[28]

Comparative surveys. A federal survey team conducts an independent survey of a home recently surveyed by a state survey agency in order to compare and contrast its findings with those of the state survey team. This comparison takes place after completion of the federal survey. When federal surveyors identify a deficiency not cited by state surveyors, they assess whether the deficiency existed at the time of the state survey and should have been cited.[29] This assessment is critical in determining whether understatement occurred, because some deficiencies cited by federal surveyors may not have existed at the time of the state survey.

Our May 2008 report stated that comparative surveys found problems at the most serious levels of noncompliance—the actual harm and immediate jeopardy levels (G through L).[30] About 15 percent of federal comparative surveys nationwide identified at least one deficiency at the G through L level that state surveyors failed to cite. While this proportion is small, CMS maintains that any missed serious deficiencies are unacceptable. Further, state surveys with understated deficiencies may allow the surveyed facilities to escape sanctions intended to discourage repeated noncompliance.

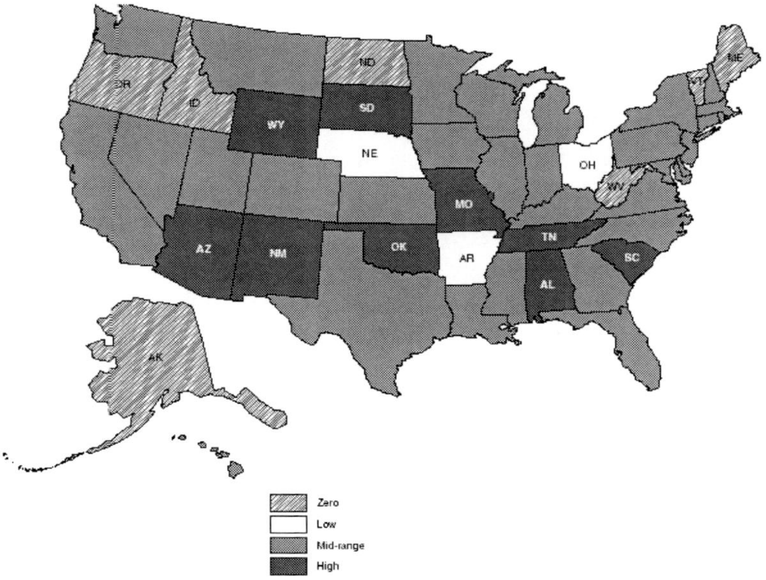

Source: GAO analysis of CMS data. Map: Copyright © Corel Corp. All rights reserved.

Note: Zero-understatement states were those that had no missed serious deficiencies on federal comparative surveys. Low-understatement states were the 10 states with the lowest percentage of missed serious deficiencies on federal comparative surveys (less than 6 percent), including all zero- understatement states. High-understatement states were the 9 states with the highest percentage of serious missed deficiencies (25 percent or more) on federal comparative surveys.

Figure 1. Zero-, Low-, and High-Understatement States, Fiscal Years 2002-2007

In our May 2008 report we found that for nine states federal surveyors identified missed serious deficiencies in 25 percent or more comparative surveys for fiscal years 2002 through 2007; we defined these states as high- understatement states (see figure 1). Zero-understatement states were states that had no federal comparative surveys identifying missed deficiencies at the actual harm or immediate jeopardy levels; and low-understatement states were the 10 states with the lowest percentage of missed serious deficiencies (less than 6 percent), including all 7 zero-understatement states.

Our May 2008 report also found that missed deficiencies at the potential for more than minimal harm level (D through F) were considerably more widespread than those at the G through L level on comparative surveys, with approximately 70 percent of comparative surveys nationwide identifying at least one missed deficiency at this level. Undetected care problems at this level are of concern because they could become more serious over time if nursing homes are not required to take corrective actions.[31]

Observational surveys. Federal surveyors accompany a state survey team to evaluate the team's performance and ability to document survey deficiencies. State teams are evaluated in six areas, including two— General Investigation and Deficiency Determination—that affect the appropriate identification and citation of deficiencies. The General Investigation segment assesses the effectiveness of state survey team actions such as collection of information, discussion of survey observations, interviews with nursing home residents, and implementation of CMS investigative protocols. The Deficiency Determination segment evaluates the skill with which the state survey teams (1) analyze and integrate all information collected, (2) use the guidance for surveyors, and (3) assess compliance with regulatory requirements. Federal observational surveys are not independent evaluations of the state survey because state surveyors may perform their survey tasks more attentively than they would if federal surveyors were not present; however, they provide more immediate feedback to state surveyors and may help identify state surveyor training needs.

We previously reported that state survey teams' poor performance on federal observational surveys in the areas of General Investigation and Deficiency Determination may contribute to the understatement of deficiencies.[32] Further, poor state performance in these two areas supported the finding of understatement as identified through the federal comparative surveys. We found that about 8 percent of state survey teams observed by federal surveyors nationwide received below-satisfactory ratings on General Investigation and Deficiency Determination from fiscal years 2002 through 2007. However, surveyors in high-understatement states performed worse in these two areas of the federal observational surveys than surveyors in the low-understatement states. For example, an average of 12 and 17 percent of state survey teams observed by federal surveyors in high-understatement states received below satisfactory ratings for these two areas, respectively. In contrast, an average of 4 percent of survey teams in low-understatement states received the same below-satisfactory scores for both deficiency determination and investigative skills.

Nationwide, one-third of nursing homes had a greater average number of serious deficiencies on federal observational surveys than on state standard surveys during fiscal years 2002 through 2007, but in eight states, it was more than half of homes. Of the one-third of homes nationwide, state standard surveys cited 83 percent fewer serious deficiencies than federal surveys during this same time period.

WEAKNESSES IN CMS SURVEY PROCESS CONTRIBUTED TO UNDERSTATEMENT, BUT LONG-TERM EFFECT OF NEW SURVEY METHODOLOGY IS NOT YET KNOWN

Over a third of both surveyors and state agency directors responding to our questionnaire identified weaknesses in the federal government's nursing home survey process that contributed to the understatement of deficiencies.[33] The weaknesses included problems with the current survey methodology; written guidance that is too long or complex; and to a lesser extent, survey predictability or other advance notice of inspections, which may allow nursing homes to conceal deficiencies. At the time our questionnaires were fielded, eight states had started implementing CMS's new survey methodology. The limited experience among these states suggests that the new methodology may improve consistency of surveys, but information is limited, and the long-term ability of the new methodology to reduce understatement is not yet known.

Weaknesses in CMS's Survey Process Contributed to Understatement

Both surveyors and state agency directors reported weaknesses in the survey process, and on our questionnaire linked these weaknesses to understatement of deficiencies. Nationally, 46 percent of nursing home surveyors responded that weaknesses in the current survey methodology resulted in missed or incorrectly identified deficiencies, with this number ranging by state from 0 to 74 percent (see table 2).[34] Thirty-six percent of state agency directors responded that weaknesses in the current survey methodology at least sometimes contributed to understatement of deficiencies in their states. One such weakness identified by both surveyors and directors was the number of survey tasks that need to be completed.

Table 2. Surveyors' and State Agency Directors' Responses to Questions on CMS's Survey Process

Questions related to CMS's survey process	Percentage of surveyors' responses	Percentage of directors' responses
Weaknesses in the current survey methodology at least sometimes result in missed or incorrectly identified deficiencies at the facility	46	36
Additional training is needed to apply CMS guidance	40	58

Source: GAO.

SURVEYOR QUOTATION ABOUT CMS WRITTEN GUIDANCE

"Appreciate the guidances and protocols. However, making Appendix PP [guidance for investigating federal quality standards] into a tome is not helping us out in the field. They are too cumbersome and voluminous. Please find a way to be more concise in these guidances."

According to surveyors and agency directors responding to our questionnaire, another weakness with the federal survey process involved CMS's written guidance to help state agencies follow federal regulations for surveying long-term care facilities.[35] Both surveyors and state agency directors mentioned concerns about the length, complexity, and subjectivity of the written guidance. One state agency director we interviewed told us that the size of the SOM made it difficult for surveyors to carry the guidance and consult it during surveys. Although the SOM is available in an electronic format, surveyors in this state did not use laptops. In addition, a small percentage of surveyors commented on our questionnaire that CMS guidance was inconsistently applied in the field. A common complaint from these surveyors was that different supervisors required different levels of evidence in order to cite a deficiency at the actual harm or immediate jeopardy level. Forty percent of surveyors and 58 percent of state agency directors reported that additional training on how to apply CMS guidance was needed.

A specific concern raised about the current survey guidance was determining the severity level for an observed deficiency. Forty-four percent of state agency directors reported on our questionnaire that confusion about CMS's definition of the actual–harm level severity requirements at least sometimes contributed to understatement in their states. CMS's guidance for determining actual harm states, "this does not include a deficient practice that only could or has caused limited consequence to the resident."[36] State agency directors from several states found this language confusing, including one director who said it is unclear whether conditions like dehydration that are reversed in the hospital should be cited as actual harm. As we reported in 2003, CMS officials acknowledged that the language linking actual harm to practices that have "limited consequences" for a resident has created confusion; however, the agency has not changed or revised this language.[37]

State agency directors and surveyors indicated that CMS's written guidance for certain federal nursing home quality standards could be improved and that revised investigative protocols were helpful.[38] Specifically, 11 state agency directors reported that CMS guidance on quality standards related to abuse could be improved. State agency directors commented that the guidance for certain quality standards was too long, with the guidance for two standards being over 50 pages long. One state agency director also noted that overly complex guidance will lead to an unmanageable survey process. Surveyors' concerns about the sufficiency of CMS's guidance varied for different quality standards (see table 3). For instance, 21 percent of surveyors nationwide reported that CMS guidance on pain management was not sufficient to identify deficiencies, whereas only 5 percent reported that guidance on pressure ulcers was not sufficient. Our analysis found that fewer surveyors had concerns with the guidance on quality standards revised through CMS's guidance update initiative.[39] For example, the guidance on pressure ulcers was revised in 2004 and the guidance on accidents was revised in 2007; these topics ranked last among the areas of concern.[40] Furthermore, state agency directors from several states commented on the usefulness of CMS's revised investigative protocols for federal quality standards.

Table 3. Percentage of Surveyors Reporting That Guidance for Certain Federal Quality Standards Was Not Sufficient to Identify Deficiencies

Federal quality standard (number)	Percentage reporting guidance on quality standard was not sufficient
Pain Management (multiple F-tags)[a, b]	21
Quality of Care / Provide Necessary Care and Services for Highest Practicable Well-Being (F-309)[c]	20
Range of Motion Mobility Treatment (F-318)	14
Accuracy of Resident Assessment (F-278)	13
Comprehensive Care Plans (F-279)	12
Sanitary Conditions for Food (F-371)[b]	12
Abuse (F-223 through F-226)[d]	11
Maintains Body Weight (F-325)[b]	11
Physical Restraints (F-221)	11
Unnecessary Drugs (F-329)[e]	11
Resident Participation in Planning Care and Treatment (F-280)	10
Accidents (F-323)[e]	8
Pressure Ulcers (F-314)[e]	5

Source: GAO.

[a] CMS consolidated guidance on pain management into F-309 on March 31, 2009.

[b] CMS revised guidance after our questionnaire of nursing home surveyors was administered in May 2008.

[c] CMS added guidance to F-309 for residents receiving hospice or dialysis services on April 10, 2009.

[d] CMS plans to begin revising guidance in Fall 2009.

[e] CMS revised guidance before our questionnaire of nursing home surveyors was administered in May 2008.

Another weakness associated with the federal survey process was the potential for surveys to be predictable based solely on their timing.[41] Eighteen percent of state agency directors reported that survey predictability or other advance notice of inspections at least sometimes contributed to understatement in their states. We analyzed state agencies' most-recent nursing home surveys and found that 29 percent of these surveys could be considered predictable due to their timing. We previously reported that survey predictability could contribute to understatement because it gives nursing homes the opportunity to conceal deficiencies if they choose to do so.[42] CMS officials previously stated that reducing survey predictability could require increased funding because more surveys would need to be conducted within 9 months of the previous survey.[43] However, CMS noted that state agencies are not funded to conduct any surveys within 9 months of the last standard survey.

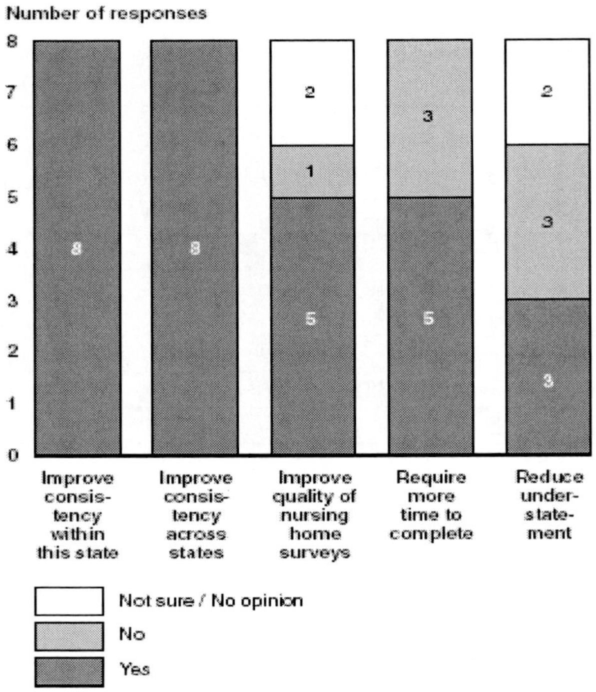

Source: GAO.

Figure 2. Eight State Agency Director Responses on Five Questions Related to the QIS

New Survey Methodology's Effect on Understatement Inconclusive

There was no consensus among the eight state agency directors who had started implementing the QIS as of November 2008 about how the new survey methodology would affect understatement.[44] Three directors reported that the QIS was likely to reduce understatement; three directors reported that it was not likely to reduce understatement; and two directors were unsure or had no opinion (see figure 2). However, all eight directors reported that the new QIS methodology was likely to improve survey consistency both within and across states. In addition, five of these directors reported that the new QIS methodology was likely to improve survey quality. Five of the eight directors also indicated that the QIS required more time than the traditional survey methodology.

CMS funded an independent evaluation of the QIS, which was completed by a contractor in December 2007.[45] The evaluation assessed the effectiveness of the new methodology by studying (1) its effect on accuracy of surveys, (2) documentation of deficiencies, (3) time required to complete survey activities, (4) number of deficiencies cited, and (5) surveyor efficiency. The evaluation did not draw a firm conclusion about the overall effectiveness of the QIS as measured through these five areas. For instance, the QIS methodology was associated with an increase in the total number of deficiencies cited, including an increase in the number of G-level deficiencies and the number of quality standard areas cited. However, the evaluation did not find that the QIS methodology increased survey accuracy, noting that QIS and traditional survey samples were comparable in overall quality and in the frequency of standards cited for deficiencies with either a pattern or widespread scope.[46] The results suggested that more deficiencies with higher scope could have been cited for both the QIS and traditional surveys. Similarly, there was no evidence that the QIS resulted in higher-quality documentation or improved surveyor efficiency. Although five state agency directors reported that the QIS required more time to complete than the traditional methodology, the evaluation found some evidence of a learning curve, suggesting that surveyors were able to complete surveys faster as they became familiar with the new process. The evaluation generated a number of recommendations for improving the QIS that are consistent with reducing understatement, such as improving the specificity and usability of investigative protocols and evaluating how well the new methodology accurately identifies the areas in which there are potential quality problems. Since the evaluation did not find improved accuracy, CMS concluded that non-QIS factors, including survey guidance clarification and surveyor training and supervision, would help improve survey accuracy. Additionally, CMS concluded that future QIS development efforts should concentrate on improving survey consistency and giving supervisors more tools to assess the performance of surveyor teams.

Ten state agency directors that had not yet started implementing the QIS responded to our questionnaire with concerns about the cost associated with implementing the new methodology, including the resources required to train staff and obtain new equipment.[47] Of these 10 directors, 3 also expressed concerns that allotting staff time for QIS implementation would prevent the agency from completing mandatory survey activities.

Workforce Shortages and Training Inadequacies May Contribute to Understatement

Workforce shortages and training inadequacies affected states' ability to complete thorough surveys, contributing to understatement of nursing home deficiencies. Responses to our questionnaires indicated that states experienced workforce shortages or were attempting to accomplish their workload with a high percentage of inexperienced surveyors. In states with fewer staff to do the work, time frames were compressed. The increased workload burden may have had an effect on the thoroughness of surveys in those states and surveyors' ability to attend training. The frequent hiring of new surveyors to address workforce shortages also burdened states' surveyor training programs. Surveyors, state agency directors, and state performance on federal observational surveys indicated that inadequacies in initial and ongoing training may have compromised survey accuracy in high-understatement states.

Workforce Shortages Sometimes Contributed to Understatement

Although a small percentage of state agency directors reported that workforce shortages always or frequently contributed to the understatement of nursing home deficiencies in their states, 36 percent indicated that workforce shortages sometimes contributed to understatement (see table 4). In many states, workforce shortages resulted in a greater reliance on inexperienced surveyors. According to state agency directors and surveyors, this collateral effect—inexperienced surveyors—also may have contributed to understatement. States also expressed concern about completing their workload, which appeared to be, in part, an outgrowth of workforce shortages and use of inexperienced surveyors.

Table 4. State Agency Directors' Responses to Questions about Surveyor Workforce Issues

	Percentage of state agency directors' responses		
How frequently do the following issues contribute to understatement in this state survey agency?	**Always/frequently**	**Sometimes**	**Infrequently/never**
Inadequate number of staff to complete thorough surveys	6	36	58
Inadequate time to complete thorough surveys	8	38	54
Reluctance to cite serious deficiencies because of workload burden	8	10	86
Inexperienced surveyors not yet comfortable with job responsibilities	16	48	34

Source: GAO.

Table 5. State Survey Agency Vacancy Rates and Percentage of State Surveyors with Less Than 2 Years' Experience

	Percentage of state agency directors' responses		
	All states	**Low-understatement states**	**High-understatement states**
Vacancy rate[a]	14	12	24
Surveyors with less than 2 years' experience[b]	30	25	38

Source: GAO.

[a] Virginia did not provide the information needed to compute a vacancy rate and it was not a high- or low-understatement state.

[b] Seven states did not report the number of surveyors with less than 2 years of experience. Among the high- and low-understatement states, only West Virginia, a low-understatement state, did not report this information.

Workforce Shortages. Since 2003, we have reported that states have experienced pervasive workforce shortages, and responses to our questionnaires indicate that shortages continue to affect states.[48] Seventy-two percent of state agency directors reported that they always or frequently had a surveyor workforce shortage, and another 16 said it occurred sometimes. The average vacancy rate for surveyors was 14 percent, and one-fourth of states had a vacancy rate of higher than 19 percent (see table 5).[49] Among the 49 reporting states, the vacancy rate ranged from a maximum of 72 percent in Alabama to 0 percent in Nevada, Rhode Island, Vermont, and Utah. The workforce shortages have stemmed mostly from the preference to employ RNs as surveyors in state survey agencies, with half of reporting states employing RNs as more than 75 percent of their surveyor workforce.[50] In the past, states have claimed that they had difficulty matching RN salaries offered by the private sector, and this hampered the hiring and retention of RNs. The Virginia state agency director commented during an interview that the nursing home industry values individuals who have passed CMS's SMQT and hires its surveyors after they are trained and certified by CMS. Virginia and others also identified the stress of the job—regular travel, time pressures to complete the workload, and the regulatory environment—as a challenge to retaining staff. Previously, we reported that workforce instability arising from noncompetitive RN surveyor salaries and hiring freezes affected states' abilities to complete their survey workload or resulted in the hiring of less-qualified staff.[51] Most recently, the poor economy has further constrained state budgets for surveyors. For example, to address its budget shortfall in 2009, California will furlough its state employees including surveyors for 2 days every month from February 2009 through June 2010.[52] An additional 11 states also reported furloughs for 2009, and 13 are considering furloughs, salary reductions, or layoffs or will employ such measures in the future.

SURVEYOR QUOTATION ABOUT INEXPERIENCED STAFF

"I have been in this department for just over 3 years, and I still do not feel comfortable with the process. I could personally use a mentor to ensure a thorough understanding of the process. I don't feel as if I can accurately identify deficiencies with the short amount of time given the survey teams to conduct surveys. I feel as if I overlook things due to trying to meet survey length time frames."

Inexperienced Surveyors. Many states are attempting to accomplish their workload with a larger share of inexperienced surveyors, and state agency directors sometimes linked this reliance on inexperienced staff to the understatement of nursing home deficiencies. On average, 30 percent of surveyors had less than 2 years' experience (see table 5); however the percentage of inexperienced surveyors ranged from 10 to 82 percent across states who reported this information.[53] Among state agency directors, 16 percent indicated that inexperienced surveyors always or frequently contributed to understatement, while another 48 percent indicated that surveyor inexperience sometimes contributed to understatement in their states. In response to our questionnaires, 26 percent of surveyors indicated that survey teams always or frequently had too many inexperienced surveyors and another 33 percent indicated that sometimes survey teams had too many inexperienced surveyors (see table 6). Half or more of all surveyors in six states—Alabama, Alaska, Arizona, Idaho, New Mexico, and Utah—reported that there were always or frequently too many new surveyors who were not yet comfortable with their job responsibilities. For example, 79 percent of surveyors in Arizona reported that too many new surveyors were not comfortable with their job responsibilities, and the state agency director was among the 34 percent who reported that survey teams sometimes had an insufficient number of experienced surveyors. Overall, 26 percent of state agency directors indicated that the skill level of surveyors has decreased in the last 5 years.

In interviews, six state agency directors commented that inexperienced surveyors possessed different skills or needed more time than experienced surveyors to complete surveys and that workforce shortages resulted in constant recruiting, over-burdened experienced surveyors, or the need for additional supervision and training resources. Four states—Kentucky, Nevada, New Mexico, and Virginia—reported not having enough dedicated training staff to handle the initial training for new surveyors.

SURVEYOR QUOTATION ABOUT INSUFFICIENT TIME TO COMPLETE SURVEYS

"Frequently G level or I/J level are not cited [due to a] lack [of] staff time."

Table 6. Surveyors' and State Agency Directors' Responses to Questions on Workforce Issues

		Percentage of responses		
Respondents	**Question**	**Always/ frequently**	**Sometimes**	**Infrequently /never**
Surveyors	**How frequently have you observed the following problems on the nursing home surveys that you have worked on?**			
	Too many new surveyors not yet comfortable with job responsibilities	26	33	35
	Survey team too small to conduct a thorough survey	21	33	42
	Survey team not given sufficient time to conduct a thorough survey	25	29	42
State Agency Directors	**In this state survey agency, how frequently do the following occur?**			
	Survey teams have a sufficient number of experienced surveyors	62	34	4
	Survey teams are sufficient size to conduct thorough surveys	74	18	8
	Survey teams are given sufficient time to conduct thorough surveys	78	16	6

Source: GAO.

Workload. State inability to complete workload was, in part, an outgrowth of the workforce shortages and reliance on inexperienced surveyors. More than two-thirds of state agency directors reported on our questionnaire that staffing posed a problem for completing complaint surveys, and more than half reported that staffing posed a problem for completing standard or revisit surveys.[54] In addition, 46 percent of state agency directors reported that time pressures always, frequently, or sometimes contributed to understatement in their states. In response to our questionnaire, 16 percent of surveyors nationwide reported that workload burden influenced the citation of deficiencies—including 14 states with 20 percent or more surveyors reporting the same. More than 50 percent of surveyors identified insufficient team size or time pressures as having an effect on the thoroughness of surveys. Surveyors' comments reiterated these concerns—over 15 percent of surveyors who wrote comments complained about the amount of time allotted to complete surveys or survey paperwork, and

11 percent indicated that staffing was insufficient to complete surveys.[55] One state agency director suggested to us that CMS establish a national team of surveyors to augment states' when they fell behind on their workload or had staffing shortages. He thought the availability of national surveyors could assist states experiencing workforce shortages and help ensure state workloads were completed. This state had experience with a similar arrangement when it hired a national contractor to complete its surveys of Intermediate Care complete its surveys of Intermediate Care Facilities for the Mentally Retarded.

Training Inadequacies May Compromise Survey Accuracy

Surveyors, state agency directors, and state performance on federal observational surveys indicated that inadequacies in initial or ongoing training may compromise the accuracy of nursing home surveys and lead to the understatement of deficiencies. In addition, workload affected surveyors' ability to attend training.

Table 7. Responses from Surveyors and State Agency Directors to Key Questions on Training

	Percentage of surveyors' responses			
	All states	Low-understatement states	High-understatement states	Percentage of directors' responses
Initial training is not sufficient:				
To ensure surveyors are able to cite appropriate scope and severity levels	24	16	29	20
To enable surveyors to identify deficiencies	26	20	28	16
Additional training is needed to:				
Interview nursing home residents	13	9	16	36[a]
Identify scope and severity levels	26	16	34	56[b]
Document deficiencies	32	27	35	62

Source: GAO.

[a] Two state agency directors did not respond to this question.

[b] One state agency director did not respond to this question.

Initial Surveyor Training. As noted earlier, even though CMS has established specific training requirements, including coursework and the SMQT certification test, states are responsible for preparing their new surveyors for the SMQT. According to CMS, 94 percent of new surveyors nationally passed the SMQT test in 2008 and, on average, surveyors answered about 77 percent of the questions correctly. These results seem to support the state agency directors' assertions that initial training was insufficient and suggest that the bar for passing the test may be set too low. Even though we cannot be certain whether the inadequacies are with the federal or state components of the training, reported differences among states in satisfaction with the initial surveyor training also could reflect gaps in state training programs. About 29 percent of surveyors in high-understatement states reported that initial training was not sufficient to cite appropriate scope and severity levels, compared with

16 percent of surveyors in low-understatement states (see table 7). Similarly, 28 percent of surveyors in high-understatement states, compared with 20 percent of those in low-understatement states, indicated that initial training was not sufficient to identify deficiencies for nursing homes. Further, 18 percent of state agency directors linked the occurrence of understatement always, frequently, or sometimes with insufficient initial training. From 16 to 20 percent of state agency directors indicated that initial training was insufficient to (1) enable surveyors to identify deficiencies and (2) assign the appropriate level of scope and severity.

Ongoing Training. Ongoing training programs are the purview of state agencies; therefore, differences between states about the sufficiency of this training also may point to gaps in the state training programs. On our questionnaire, about 34 percent of surveyors in high-understatement states indicated a need for additional training on (1) identifying appropriate scope and severity levels and (2) documenting deficiencies. This was significantly more than those from low-understatement states, which indicated less of a need for additional training in these areas—16 and 27 percent, respectively. Among state agency directors, 10 percent attributed understatement always or frequently to insufficient ongoing training, while 14 percent indicated that insufficient ongoing training sometimes gave rise to understatement. Although 74 percent of state agency directors indicated that the state had ongoing annual training requirements, the required number of hours and the type of training varied widely by state in 2007. Among the 33 states that provided the required amount of annual state training, these hours ranged from 0 to 120 hours per year. Meanwhile, 37 states reported one or more type of required training: 32 states required surveyors to attend periodic training, 22 required on-the-job training, 10 required online computerized training, and 13 states required some other type of training.

State agency directors indicated that they relied on CMS materials for ongoing training of experienced surveyors, yet many reported additional training needs and suggested that use of electronic media could make continuing education and new guidance more accessible. While 98 percent of states indicated that the CMS written guidance materials and resources were useful, over 50 percent of all state agency directors identified additional training needs in documenting deficiencies, citing deficiencies at the appropriate scope and severity level, and applying CMS guidance. On federal observational surveys, an average of 17 to 12 percent of survey teams in high-understatement states received below-satisfactory ratings for Deficiency Determination and General Investigation, respectively—two skills critical for preventing understatement. In contrast, an average of 4 percent of survey teams in low-understatement states received the same below-satisfactory scores for both deficiency determination and investigative skills. Furthermore, of the 476 surveyors who commented about training needs, one-quarter indicated a need for training support from either CMS or state agencies; and between 12 to 7 percent of those who commented on training needs identified topics such as: documenting deficiencies, identifying scope and severity, CMS guidance, and medical knowledge.[56]

Inability to Attend Training. States' workload requirements and workforce shortages affected the surveyors' ability to attend initial and ongoing training. Seven of the eight state agency directors we interviewed linked workforce shortages and resource constraints to their state's ability to complete the survey workload or allow staff to participate in training courses. One director stated that workload demands compromised comprehensive training for new staff, and another reported difficulty placing new staff in CMS's initial training programs. Due to workload demands, a third state agency director stated that she could not allow experienced staff time away from surveying to attend training courses even when staff paid their own way. Five of the seven state agency directors suggested that it would be more efficient for training activities to be conducted more locally such as in their states or to be available through online, video, or other electronic media, and several emphasized the need to reduce or eliminate travel for training. Although four states also expressed a preference for interactive training opportunities, one state believed that technological solutions could allow for more accessible training that was also interactive.

State Supervisory Reviews Often Are Not Designed to Identify Understatement

State supervisory reviews, which generally occurred more frequently on higher-level deficiencies, often are not designed to identify understated deficiencies. State agencies generally conducted more supervisory reviews on surveys with higher-level deficiencies, compared to surveys with deficiencies at the potential for more than minimal harm level (D through F)—the deficiencies most likely to be understated. While focus on higher- level deficiencies enables states to be certain that such deficiencies are well documented, not reviewing surveys with deficiencies at lower levels represents a missed opportunity to ensure that all serious deficiencies are cited. State surveyors who reported having frequent changes made to their survey reports during supervisory reviews also more often reported they were burdened by other factors contributing to understatement, such as workforce shortages and survey methodology weaknesses.

Supervisory Reviews Often Focused on Higher-Level Deficiencies

According to state agency directors' responses to our questionnaire, states generally focused supervisory review on surveys with higher-level deficiencies, rather than on the surveys with deficiencies at the potential for more than minimal-harm level (D through F)—the deficiencies most likely to be understated. During supervisory reviews, either direct-line supervisors or central state agency staff may review draft survey records.[57] On average, surveys at the D through F level underwent about two steps of review, while surveys with deficiencies at the immediate jeopardy level (J through L) went through three steps.[58] For example, Washington reviews its surveys using either a two-step review that includes survey team and field manager reviews or a three-step process that includes both these reviews and an additional review by central state agency staff for serious deficiencies. As a result, central state agency staff in Washington do not review deficiencies below the level of actual harm. In addition we found that five states—Alaska, Hawaii, Illinois, Nebraska, and Nevada— did not review all surveys with deficiencies at the D through F levels. In fact, Hawaii did not report supervisory review of deficiencies at any level (see figure 3).[59] It is difficult to know if additional supervisory reviews—the second, third, or fourth review—help make survey records more accurate and less likely to be understated, or if these reviews result in more frequent changes to deficiency citations. However, if deficiency citations with the potential for more than minimal-harm level (D through F) are not reviewed, states miss the opportunity to assess whether these deficiencies warrant a higher-level citation, for example, the level of actual harm or immediate jeopardy.

Because a majority of states are organized into geographically-based district or regional offices, review by central state agency staff, particularly quality assurance staff, is critical to help ensure consistency and detect understatement. However, 26 states reported that no central state agency staff reviews were conducted for surveys with deficiencies at the potential for more than minimal harm (D through F). These results are consistent with a finding from our 2003 report—that half of the 16 states we contacted for that report did not have a quality assurance process to help ensure that the scope and severity of less serious deficiencies were not understated.[60]

According to most of the eight state officials we interviewed, supervisory reviews commonly focused on documentation principles or evidentiary support, not on reducing understatement. For example, all eight states used supervisory reviews to assess the accuracy and strength of the evidence surveyors used to support deficiency citations, and three of these states reported that they emphasized reviewing survey records for documentation principles. Furthermore, seven out of eight states indicated that surveys with serious deficiencies—those that may be subject to enforcement proceedings—went through additional steps of review compared with surveys citing deficiencies with the potential for more than minimal harm (D through F).

Reports of Changes to Deficiencies during Supervisory Reviews May Be Related to Other Factors That Contribute to Understatement

Surveyor reports of changes to deficiency citations during supervisory reviews may be related to other factors the state is experiencing that also contribute to understatement, such as workforce shortages and survey methodology weaknesses.

Surveyor Quotation about Supervisory Review

"We have problems at times with nonclinical supervisors and district managers, [and with] a past branch chief not understanding clinical issues and thus not supporting surveyor findings. We've had deficiencies tossed out for surveys and IDR deficiencies deleted, not for lack of documentation, but for lack of understanding of the issues involved."

Changes to Deficiencies. Fifty-four percent of surveyors nationwide reported on our questionnaire that supervisors at least sometimes removed the deficiency that was cited, and 53 percent of surveyors noted that supervisors at least sometimes changed the scope and severity level of cited deficiencies. Of the surveyors, who reported that supervisors sometimes removed deficiencies, 13 percent reported that supervisors always or frequently removed deficiencies—including 12 states with 20 percent or more of their surveyors reporting that deficiencies were removed.

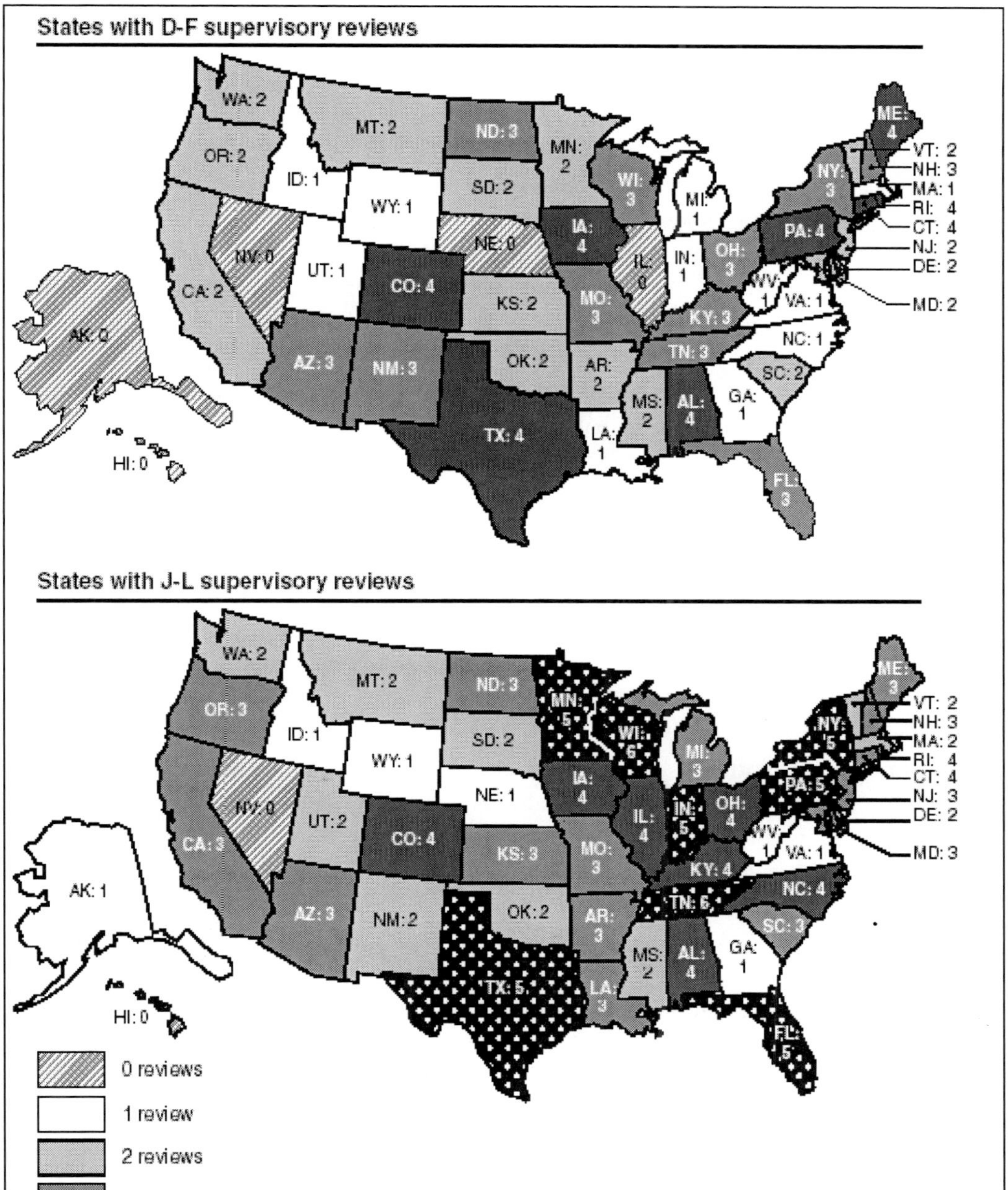

Note: Hawaii did not report conducting supervisory reviews. Forty states review a sample of all draft surveys. Such reviews may include additional examination of surveys with deficiencies at either the D through F or J through L levels.

Figure 3. Number of State Supervisory Reviews at the Potential for More than Minimal Harm (D-F) and Immediate Jeopardy Levels (J-L)

Surveyor reports of changes in deficiency citations alone make it difficult to know whether the original deficiency citation or the supervisor's revised citation was a more accurate reflection of a nursing home's quality of care. Additionally, there are many reasons that survey records might be changed during supervisory review. When a surveyor fails to provide sufficient evidence for deficient practices, it may be difficult to tell whether the deficiency was not appropriately cited or if the surveyor did not collect all the available evidence. Kentucky's state agency director offered one possible explanation—that changes to surveys often reflected a need for more support for the deficiencies cited, such as additional evidence from observations. Nevada's state agency director stated that changes to survey records occurred when it was often too late to gather more evidence in support of deficiencies.

Surveyors who reported that supervisors frequently changed deficiencies also more often reported experiencing other factors that contribute to understatement. We found associations between surveyor reports of changes to deficiencies and workforce shortages and survey methodology weaknesses.

- **Workforce shortages.** Surveyors reporting workforce shortages, including survey teams with too many new surveyors and survey teams that were either too small or given insufficient time to conduct thorough surveys, more often also reported that supervisors frequently removed deficiencies or changed the scope and severity of deficiency citations during supervisory reviews.

- **Survey methodology weaknesses.** Surveyors reporting weaknesses in the current survey methodology more often also reported that supervisors frequently removed deficiencies or changed the scope and severity of deficiency citations during supervisory reviews.

- **Supervisory Reviews and Understatement.** In certain cases, survey agency directors and state performance on federal comparative surveys linked supervisory reviews to understatement. Twenty-two percent of state agency directors attributed inadequate supervisory review processes to understatement in their states at least sometimes.[61] In addition, significant differences existed between zero-understatement states and all other states, including high-understatement states, in the percentage of surveyors reporting frequent changes to citations during supervisory reviews. Only about 4 percent of surveyors in zero-understatement states reported that citations were always or frequently removed or changed and that the scope and severity cited were changed, while about 12 percent of surveyors in all other states indicated the same (see table 8). To address concerns with supervisory reviews, Nevada recently reduced its process from two steps to a single step review by survey team supervisors to address surveyor complaints about changes made during supervisory reviews.

In addition, we observed a relationship between state practices to notify surveyors of changes made during supervisory reviews and surveyor reports of deficiency removal and explanation of changes. Specifically, compared to surveyors in states that require supervisors to notify surveyors of changes made during supervisory review, surveyors from states where no notification is required reported more often that supervisors removed deficiencies and less often that explanations for these changes, when given, were reasonable.

Similarly, we found an association between the frequency of explained and reasonable changes and zero-understatement states, possibly demonstrating the positive effect of practices to notify surveyors of changes made during supervisory reviews. Nursing home surveyors from zero-understatement states more often reported that supervisors explained changes and that their explanations seemed reasonable compared to surveyors in all other states. State agency directors in Massachusetts and New Mexico stated that explanations of changes to the survey record provided opportunities for one-on-one feedback to surveyors and discussions about deficiencies being removed.

State Agency Practices and External Pressure May Compromise Survey Accuracy and Lead to Understatement in a Few States

Nursing home surveyors and state agency directors in a minority of states told us that in isolated cases issues such as a state agency practice of noncitation, external pressure from the nursing home industry, and an unbalanced IDR process may have led to the understatement of deficiencies. In a few states, surveyors more often identified problems with noncitation practices and IDR processes compared to state agency directors. Yet, a few state agency directors acknowledged either noncitation practices, external pressure, or an IDR process that favored nursing home operators over resident welfare. Although not all the issues raised by surveyors were corroborated by the state agency directors in their states, surveyor reports clustered in a few states gives credence to the notion that such conditions may lead to understatement.

Table 8. Percentage of Surveyors Reporting Changes in Deficiency Citations during Supervisory Review

	Percentage of surveyors' responses	
	Zero-understatement states	**All other states**
Surveyors reporting that:		
Supervisors always or frequently remove or change deficiency cited	5	13
Supervisors always or frequently changed the scope and severity cited	4	12

Source: GAO.

Surveyors Reported Noncitation Practices in a Small Number of States

Approximately 20 percent of surveyors nationwide and over 40 percent of surveyors in five states reported that their state agency had at least one of the following noncitation practices: (1) not citing certain deficiencies, (2) not citing deficiencies above a certain scope and severity level, and (3) allowing nursing homes to correct deficiencies without receiving a citation (see figure 4). Only four state agency directors acknowledged the existence of such practices in their states on our questionnaire and only one of these directors was from the five states most often identified by surveyors. One of these directors commented on our questionnaire that one of these practices occurs only in "rare individual cases." Another director commented that a particular federal quality standard is not related to patient outcome and therefore should not be cited above a Level F. According to CMS protocols, when noncompliance with a federal requirement has been identified, the state agency should cite all deficiencies associated with the noncompliance. CMS regional officials we interviewed were not aware of any current statewide noncitation practices.[62]

SURVEYOR QUOTATION ABOUT STATE NONCITATION PRACTICES

"I have been criticized by my supervisor on more than one occasion for citing too many deficiencies at facilities [that] have an ongoing history of repeat tags from survey to survey and many complaints surveys between annual surveys. My supervisor states that citing too many deficiencies 'confuses' the facility and creates a 'hostile' environment."

Not citing certain deficiencies. Nationally, 9 percent of surveyors reported a state agency practice that surveyors not cite certain deficiencies. However, in four states over 30 percent of surveyors reported their state agency had this noncitation practice, including over 60 percent of New Mexico surveyors. In some cases, surveyors reported receiving direct instructions from supervisors not to cite certain deficiencies. In other cases, surveyors' reports of noncitation practices may have been based on their interpretation of certain management practices. For instance, surveyors commented that some state agency practices—such as providing inadequate time to observe and document deficiencies or frequently deleting deficiency citations during supervisory review— seemed like implicit or indirect leadership from the agency to avoid citing deficiencies. One state agency director we interviewed agreed that surveyors may report the existence of noncitation practices when their citations are changed during supervisory review. This official told us that when surveyors' deficiencies are deleted or downgraded, the surveyors may choose not to cite similar deficiencies in the future because they perceive being overruled as an implicit state directive not to cite those deficiencies.

Not citing deficiencies above a certain scope and severity level. Although nationwide less than 8 percent of surveyors reported a state agency practice that surveyors not cite deficiencies above a certain scope and severity level, in two states over 25 percent of surveyors reported that their state agency used this type of noncitation practice. One reason state agencies might use this noncitation practice could be to help manage the agency's workload. In particular, citing deficiencies at a lower scope and severity might help the agency avoid additional work associated with citing higher-level deficiencies, such as survey revisits or IDR.[63] In one of the two states mentioned above, 54 percent of surveyors indicated that the workload burden influenced their citations. Additionally, as we described earlier, 16 percent of surveyors nationwide indicated that workload burden influenced the citation of deficiencies and more than half of state agency directors (including those from the two states mentioned above) responded that staffing was not sufficient to complete revisit surveys. While our questionnaire focused on not citing deficiencies above a certain scope and severity level, a few surveyors commented on being discouraged from citing lower-level deficiencies due to time pressures to complete surveys. Agency officials in two states told us that surveyors may miss some deficiencies due to limited survey time and resources.

Allowing nursing homes to correct deficiencies without citing them on the survey record. Nationwide, approximately 12 percent of surveyors reported this type of noncitation practice. However, in five states, at least 30 percent of surveyors reported their state agency allowed nursing homes to correct deficiencies without citing those deficiencies on the official survey record. Comments from surveyors suggest that state agencies may use this type of practice to avoid actions that nursing homes or the industry would dispute or interpret as excessive. Similarly, several surveyors commented that they were instructed to cite only one deficiency for a single type of negative outcome, even when more than one problem existed. However, CMS guidance requires state agencies to cite all problems that lead to a negative outcome. The decrease in G-level citations that occurred after CMS implemented the double G immediate sanctions policy in January 2000 also suggests that some states may have avoided citing deficiencies that would result in enforcement actions for the nursing home.[64] The total number of G-level deficiency citations nationwide dropped from approximately 10,000 in 1999 to 7,700 in 2000.[65]

State Agency Directors in a Few States Reported That External Pressure Contributed to Understatement

State agency directors from 12 states reported experiencing external pressure from at least one of the following stakeholder groups: (1) the nursing home surveyed, (2) the nursing home industry, or (3) state or federal legislators. Examples of such external pressure include pressure to reduce federal or state nursing home regulation or to delete specific deficiencies cited by the state agency. Of the 12 state agency directors, 7 reported that external pressure at least sometimes contributed to the understatement of deficiencies in their states, while the other 5 indicated that it infrequently or never contributed to understatement.

SURVEYOR QUOTATION ABOUT EXTERNAL PRESSURE

"The larger corporations often pressure our [state agency] Central Office to change and delete citations. Our Central Office changes not only wording but content and intent of the citation, when they were not on site. There is a great deal of political push and pull—the interference from State Senators and Representatives protecting their re-electability and not the rights of the residents (who don't vote)."

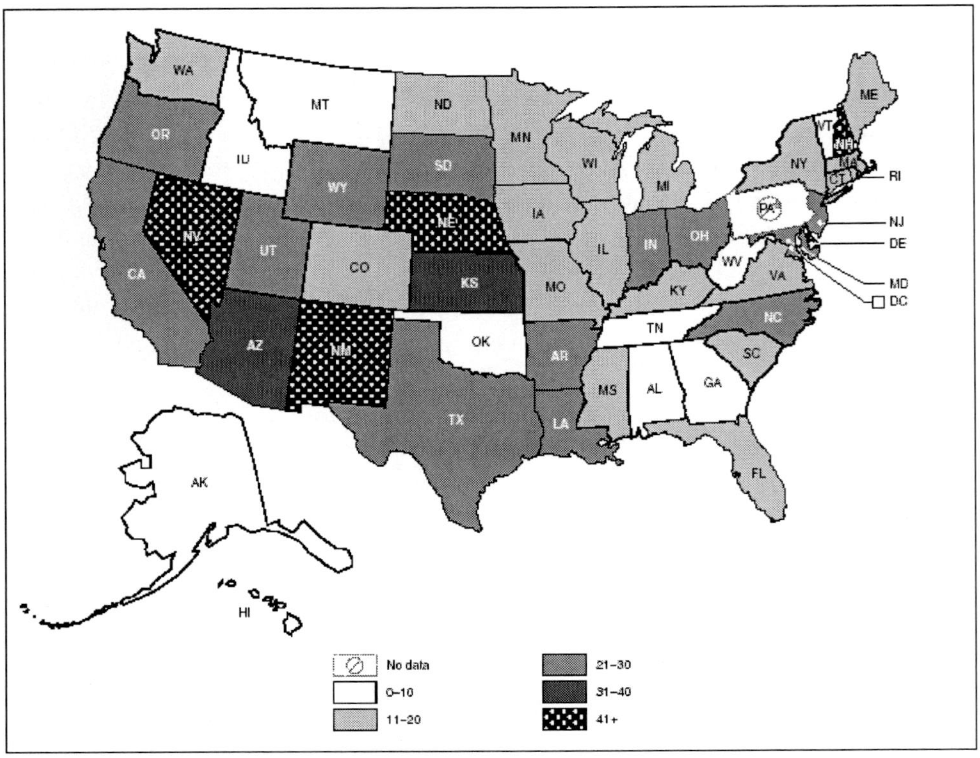

[a] Responses from Pennsylvania surveyors could not be included because the state agency directed nursing home surveyors not to respond to our questionnaire.

Figure 4. Percentage of Surveyors in Each State Reporting at Least One Noncitation Practice

Adversarial attitude toward nursing home surveys. Two states we interviewed—State A and State B—commented on the adversarial attitude that industry and legislative representatives had toward nursing home surveys at times.[66] For instance, state agency officials from State A told us that the state nursing home association organized several forums to garner public and legislative support for curtailing state regulation of facilities. According to officials in this state, the influential industry groups threatened to request legislation to move the state agency to a different department and to deny the confirmation of the director's gubernatorial appointment if the citations of G level or higher deficiencies increased. CMS regional office officials responsible for State A told us that the state may be experiencing more intense external pressure this year given the current economy, because providers have greater concerns about the possible financial implications of deficiency citations—fines or increased insurance rates.

Similarly, officials from State B told us that when facilities are close to termination, the state agency receives phone calls from state delegates questioning the agency's survey results. Officials from State B also told us that the Governor's office instructed the state agency not to recommend facilities for enforcement actions. Officials from the CMS regional office responsible for State B told us that this situation was not problematic because CMS was ultimately responsible for determining enforcement actions based on deficiency citations. However, this regional office's statement is inconsistent with (1) language in the SOM that calls for states to recommend enforcement actions to the regional office, and (2) assertions from the regional office responsible for State A that it infrequently disagrees with state recommendations for sanctions. A third state agency director commented that the agency had been called before state legislative committees in 2007-2008 to defend deficiency citations that led to the termination of facilities. A fourth state agency director also commented on our questionnaire that legislators had pressured the state agency on behalf of nursing homes to get citations reduced or eliminated and prevent enforcement actions for the facilities. In addition, a few surveyors commented that at times when nursing homes were unhappy with their survey results the homes or their state legislators would ask state agency management to remove the citations from the survey record, resulting in the deletion or downgrading of deficiencies. Further, comments from a few surveyors indicated that they may steer clear of citing deficiencies when they perceive the citation might cause a home to complain or exert pressure for changes in the survey record.

Interference in the survey process. In a few cases, external pressure appeared to directly interfere with the nursing home survey process. State agency officials from two states—State A and an additional fifth state— reported that state legislators or industry representatives had appeared on- site during nursing home surveys. Although in some cases the legislators just observed the survey process, officials from these two states explained that third parties also have interfered with the process by questioning or intimidating surveyors. The state agency director from the fifth state commented on our questionnaire that the nursing home industry sent legal staff on-site during surveys to interfere with the survey process. Similarly, officials from State A told us that during one survey, a home's lawyer was on-site reviewing nursing home documentation before surveyors were given access to these documents. Officials from State A also told us that state legislators have attended surveys to question surveyors about their work and whether state agency executives were coercing them to find deficiencies. We discussed this issue with the CMS regional officials responsible for State A, who acknowledged that this type of interference had occurred.

States' need for support from CMS. In the face of significant external pressure, officials from States A and B suggested that they need support from CMS; however, CMS regional office officials did not always acknowledge external pressure reported by the states. This year, State A terminated a survey due to significant external pressure from a nursing home and requested that the CMS regional office complete the revisit survey for them. Six weeks later, the federal team completed the survey and found many of the same problems that this state team had previously identified before it stopped the survey. Officials from State A suggested the need for other support as well, such as creating a federal law that would require state agencies to report external pressure and ensure whistleblower protections for state officials who report pressure and allowing sanctions for inappropriate conduct. CMS officials from the regional office responsible for State A stated that external pressure might indirectly contribute to understatement by increasing surveyor mistakes from the additional stress, workload, focus on documentation, and supervisory reviews. Conversely, CMS regional officials did not acknowledge that State B experienced external pressure and officials from State B thought that CMS should be more consistent in its requirements and enforcement actions.

Unbalanced IDR Processes Might Have Contributed to Understatement in a Few States

States with unbalanced IDR processes may experience more understatement. IDR processes vary across states in structure, volume of proceedings, and resulting changes. According to state agency directors' responses to our questionnaire, 16 IDRs were requested per 100 homes in fiscal year 2007, with this number ranging among states from 0 to 57 per 100 homes.[67] For IDRs occurring in fiscal year 2007, 20 percent of disputed deficiencies were deleted and 7 percent were downgraded in scope or severity, but in four states, at least 40 percent of disputed deficiencies were deleted through this process.[68] CMS does not provide protocols on how states should operate their IDR processes, leaving IDR operations to state survey agencies' discretion. For example, states may choose to conduct IDR meetings in writing, by telephone, or through face-to-face conferences. State agencies also have the option to involve outside entities, including legal representation, in their IDR operations.

On the basis of responses from surveyors and state agency directors clustered in a few states, problems with the IDR processes—such as frequent hearings, deficiencies that are frequently deleted or downgraded through the IDR process, or outcomes that favor nursing home operators over resident welfare—may have contributed to the understatement of deficiencies in those states. Although reports of such problems were not common—only 16 percent of surveyors nationwide reported on our questionnaire that their state's IDR process favored nursing home operators—in four states over 40 percent of surveyors reported that their IDR process favored nursing home operators (see fig. 5), including one state where a substantial percentage of surveyors identified at least one noncitation practice. While only one state agency director reported that the IDR process favored nursing home operators, three other directors acknowledged that frequent IDR hearings at least sometimes contributed to the understatement of deficiencies. For example, in some states surveyors may hesitate to cite deficiencies that they believe will be disputed by the nursing home.

SURVEYOR QUOTATION ABOUT THE IDR PROCESS

"The IDR process is inconsistent. Over the years we have been on all ends of the spectrum—between having involved panels who have an understanding of the survey process versus people who know nothing about the process and have no idea how to apply the federal regulations. (The latter is the current make-up.) When we have a panel made up of the latter, the word spreads throughout the state and there is a very large increase in requests for IDR. The reason is that this type of panel tends to delete most everything for 'insufficient evidence' but cannot coherently explain how they came [to] that decision."

In isolated cases, a lack of balance with the IDR process appeared to be a result of external pressure. In one state, the state agency director reported that the nursing home industry sent association representatives to the IDR, which increased the contentiousness of the process.

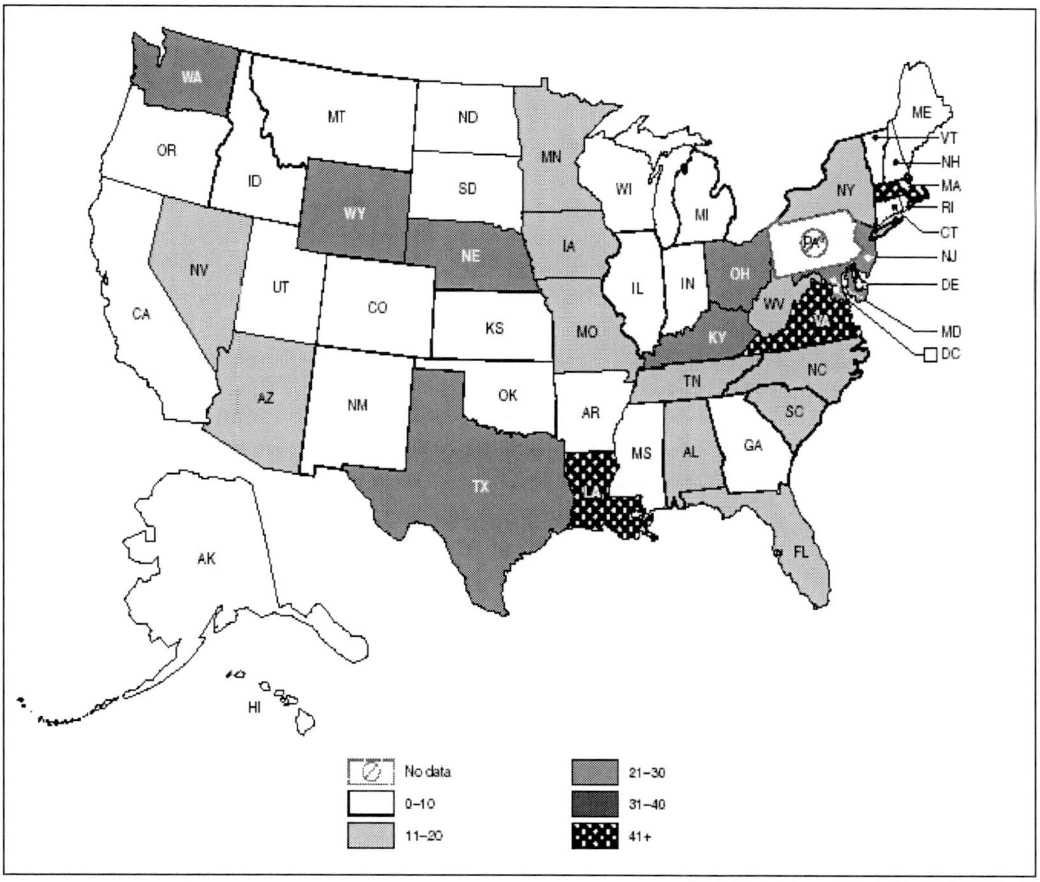

Source: GAO. Map: Copyright © Corel Corp. All rights reserved.

[a] Responses from Pennsylvania surveyors could not be included because the state agency directed nursing home surveyors not to respond to our questionnaire.

Figure 5. Percentage of Surveyors in Each State Reporting the IDR Process Favored Concerns of Nursing Home Operators over Resident Welfare

In another state, officials told us that a large nursing home chain worked with the state legislature to set up an alternative to the state IDR process, which has been used only by facilities in this chain. Through this alternative appeals process, both the state agency and the nursing home have legal representation, and compliance decisions are made by an adjudicator. According to agency officials in this state, the adjudicators for this alternative appeals process do not always have health care backgrounds. While CMS gives states the option to allow outside entities to conduct the IDR, the states should maintain ultimate responsibility for IDR decisions. [69] CMS regional officials stated it would not consider the outcome of this alternative appeals process when assessing deficiencies or determining enforcement actions. Regardless, these actions may have affected surveyors' perceptions of the balance of the states' IDRs, because over twice the national average of surveyors in this state reported that their IDR process favored nursing home operators.

CONCLUSIONS

Reducing understatement is critical to protecting the health and safety of vulnerable nursing home residents and ensuring the credibility of the survey process. Federal and state efforts will require a sustained, longterm commitment because understatement arises from weaknesses in several interrelated areas—including CMS's survey process, surveyor workforce and training, supervisory review processes, and state agency practices and external pressure.

- **Concerns about CMS's Survey Process.** Survey methodology and guidance are integral to reliable and consistent state nursing home surveys, and we found that weaknesses in these areas were linked to understatement by both surveyors and state agency directors. Both groups reported struggling to interpret existing guidance, and differences in interpretation were linked to understatement, especially in determining what constitutes actual harm. Surveyors noted that the current survey guidance was too lengthy, complex, and subjective. Additionally, they had fewer concerns about care areas for which CMS has issued revised interpretive protocols. In its development of the QIS, CMS has taken steps to revise the nursing home survey methodology. However, development and implementation of the QIS in a small group of states has taken approximately 10 years, and full implementation of the new methodology is not expected to be completed until 2014. The experience of the QIS was mixed regarding improvement in the quality of surveys, and the independent evaluation generated a number of recommendations for improving the QIS. CMS concluded that it needed to focus future QIS development efforts on improving survey consistency and giving supervisors more tools to assess performance of surveyor teams.

- **Ongoing Workforce and Surveyor Training Challenges.** Workforce shortages in state survey agencies increase the need for high-quality initial and ongoing training for surveyors. Currently, high vacancy rates can place pressure on state surveyors to complete surveys under difficult circumstances, including compressed time frames, inadequately staffed survey teams, and too many inexperienced surveyors. States are responsible for hiring and retaining surveyors and have grappled with pervasive and intractable workforce shortages. State agency directors struggling with these workforce issues reported the need for more readily accessible training for both their new and experienced surveyors that did not involve travel to a central location. Nearly 30 percent of surveyors in high-understatement states stated that initial surveyor training, which is primarily a state activity that incorporates two CMS on-line computer courses and a 1-week federal basic training course culminating in the SMQT, was not adequate to identify deficiencies and cite them at the appropriate scope and severity level. State agency directors reported that workforce shortages also impede states' ability to provide ongoing training opportunities for experienced staff and that additional CMS online training and electronic training media would help states maintain an experienced, well-informed workforce. They noted that any such support should be cognizant of states' current resource constraints, including limited funding of travel for training.

- **Supervisory Review Limitations.** Currently, CMS provides little guidance on how states should structure supervisory review processes, leaving the scope of this important quality-assurance tool exclusively to the states and resulting in considerable variation throughout the nation in how these processes are structured. We believe that state quality assurance processes are a more effective preventive measure against understatement because they have the potential to be more immediate and cover more surveys than the limited number of federal comparative surveys conducted in each state. However, compared to reviews of serious deficiencies, states conducted relatively fewer reviews of deficiencies at the D through F level, those that were most frequently understated throughout the nation, to assess whether or not such deficiencies were cited at too low a scope and severity level. In addition, we found that frequent changes to survey results made during supervisory review were symptomatic of workforce shortages and survey methodology weaknesses. For example, surveyors who reported that survey teams had too many new surveyors, more often also reported either frequent changes to or removals of deficiencies during supervisory reviews—indicating that states with inexperienced workforces may rely more heavily on supervisory reviews. In addition, variation existed in the type of feedback surveyors receive when deficiencies are changed or removed during supervisory reviews, providing surveyors with inconsistent access to valuable feedback and training. CMS did not implement our previous recommendation to require states to have a quality assurance process that includes, at a minimum, a review of a sample of survey reports below the actual harm level to assess the appropriateness of the scope and severity cited and help reduce understatement.

- **State Agency Practices and External Pressure.** In a few states, noncitation practices, challenging relationships with the industry or legislators, or unbalanced IDR processes—those that surveyors regard as favoring nursing home operators over resident welfare—may have had a negative effect on survey quality and resulted in the citation of fewer nursing home deficiencies than was warranted. In one state, both the state agency director and over 40 percent of surveyors acknowledged the existence of a noncitation practice such as allowing a home to correct a deficiency without receiving a citation. Forty percent of surveyors in four other states also responded on our questionnaire that noncitation practices existed. Currently, CMS does not explicitly address such practices in its guidance to states, and its oversight is limited to reviews of citation patterns, feedback from state surveyors, state performance reviews, and federal monitoring surveys to determine if such practices exist. Twelve state agency directors reported on our questionnaire experiencing some kind of external pressure. For example, in one state a legislator attended a survey and questioned surveyors as to whether state agency executives were coercing them to find deficiencies. Under such circumstances, it is difficult to know if the affected surveyors are consistently enforcing federal standards and reporting all deficiencies at the appropriate scope and severity levels. States' differing experiences regarding the enforcement of federal standards and collaboration with their CMS regional offices in the face of significant external pressure also may confuse or undermine a thorough and independent survey process. If surveyors believe that CMS does not fully or consistently support the enforcement of federal standards, these surveyors may choose to avoid citing deficiencies that they perceive may trigger a reaction from external stakeholders. In addition, deficiency determinations may be influenced when IDR processes are perceived to favor nursing home operators over resident welfare.

Because many aspects of federal and state operations contribute to the understatement of deficiencies on nursing home surveys, mitigating this problem will require the concerted effort of both entities. The interrelated nature of these challenges suggests a need for increased CMS attention on the areas noted above and additional federal support for states' efforts to enforce federal nursing home quality standards.

Recommendations for Executive Action

To address concerns about weaknesses in CMS survey methodology and guidance, we recommend that the Administrator of CMS take the following two actions:

- make sure that action is taken to address concerns identified with the new QIS methodology, such as ensuring that it accurately identifies potential quality problems; and
- clarify and revise existing CMS written guidance to make it more concise, simplify its application in the field, and reduce confusion, particularly on the definition of actual harm.

  To address surveyor workforce shortages and insufficient training, we recommend that the Administrator of CMS take the following two actions:
- consider establishing a pool of additional national surveyors that could augment state survey teams or identify other approaches to help states experiencing workforce shortages;
- evaluate the current training programs and division of responsibility between federal and state components to determine the most cost- effective approach to: (1) providing initial surveyor training to new surveyors, and (2) supporting the continuing education of experienced surveyors.

  To address inconsistencies in state supervisory reviews, we recommend that the Administrator of CMS take the following action:
- set an expectation through guidance that states have a supervisory review program as a part of their quality-assurance processes that includes routine reviews of deficiencies at the level of potential for more than minimal harm (D-F) and that provides feedback to surveyors regarding changes made to citations.

  To address state agency practices and external pressure that may compromise survey accuracy, we recommend that the Administrator of CMS take the following two actions:

- reestablish expectations through guidance to state survey agencies that noncitation practices—official or unofficial—are inappropriate, and systematically monitor trends in states' citations; and
- establish expectations through guidance to state survey agencies to communicate and collaborate with their CMS regional offices when they experience significant pressure from legislators or the nursing home industry that may affect the survey process or surveyors' perceptions.

AGENCY AND AHFSACOMMENTS AND OUR EVALUATION

We provided a draft of this chapter to HHS and AHFSA for comment. In response, the Acting Administrator of CMS provided written comments. CMS noted that the report adds value to important public policy discussions regarding the survey process and contributes ideas for solutions on the underlying potential causes of understatement. CMS fully endorsed five of our seven recommendations and indicated it would explore alternate solutions to our remaining two recommendations, one of which the agency did not plan to implement on a national scale. (CMS's comments are reprinted in appendix II.) AHFSA's comments noted that several states agreed with one of our recommendations, but did not directly express agreement or disagreement with the other recommendations. AHFSA made several other comments on our findings and recommendations as summarized below.

CMS

CMS agreed with five of our recommendations that called for: (1) addressing issues identified with the new QIS methodology, (2)evaluating current training programs, (3) setting expectations that states have a supervisory review program, (4) reestablishing expectations that noncitation practices are inappropriate, and (5) establishing expectations that states communicate with their CMS regional office when they experience significant pressure from legislators or the nursing home industry. In its comments, the agency cited several ongoing efforts as mechanisms for addressing some of our recommendations. While we acknowledge the importance of these ongoing efforts, in some areas we believe more progress and investigation are likely needed to fully address our findings and recommendations. For example, we recommended that CMS ensure that measures are taken to address issues identified with the new QIS methodology, such as ensuring that it accurately identifies potential quality problems; CMS's response cited Desk Audit Reports that enable supervisors to provide improved feedback to surveyors and quarterly meetings of a user group as evidence of efforts under way to continuously improve the QIS and to increase survey consistency. However, we noted that a 2007 evaluation of the QIS did not find improved survey accuracy compared to the traditional survey process and recommended that CMS evaluate how well the QIS accurately identifies areas in which there were potential quality problems. While improving the consistency of the survey process is important, CMS must also focus on addressing the accuracy of QIS surveys.

For the remaining two recommendations, CMS described alternative solutions that it indicated the agency would explore:

- *Guidance.* The agency agreed in principle with our recommendation to clarify and revise existing written guidance to make it more concise, simplify its application in the field, and reduce confusion. However, CMS disagreed with shortening the guidance as the preferred method for achieving such clarification. Instead, the agency suggested an alternative— the creation of some short reference documents for use in the field that contain cross-links back to the full guidance—that we believe would fulfill the intent of our recommendation.

- *National surveyor pool.* CMS indicated it did not plan to implement our recommendation to consider establishing a pool of additional national surveyors that could augment state survey teams experiencing workforce shortages, at least not on a national scale. The agency stated that the establishment of national survey teams was problematic for several reasons, including that it (1) began to blur the line between state accountability for meeting performance expectations and compensating states for problematic performance due to state management decisions, and (2) was improper for CMS to tell states how to make personnel decisions While the agency noted that it used national contractors to perform surveys for other types of facilities such as organ transplant centers, it expressed concern about their use to compensate for state performance issues because of the more frequent nursing home surveys.

We believe that state workforce shortages are a separate issue from state performance on surveys. Since 2003, we have reported pervasive state workforce shortages and this chapter confirms that such shortages continue.[70] For example, we reported that one-fourth of states had vacancy rates higher than 19 percent and that one state reported a 72 percent vacancy rate. We also believe that addressing workforce shortages is critical to creating an effective system of oversight for nursing homes and reducing understatement throughout the nation.

However, CMS noted that it would explore this issue with a state-federal work group in order to identify any circumstances in which a national pool may be advisable and to identify any additional solutions. Reflecting this comment from CMS, we have revised our original recommendation to include other potential solutions as well as a national pool of surveyors. One suggestion in AHFSA comments may be worth exploring in this regard—providing funds to state survey agencies for recruitment and retention activities.

AHFSA

AHFSA commented that vigorous oversight and enforcement are essential to improving the quality of life and quality of care for health care consumers and are critical if improvements already achieved are to be maintained. The association noted that several states agreed with our recommendation on the need for CMS to revise existing written guidance to make it more concise. While the association did not directly express agreement or disagreement with our other recommendations, it did note that most states would need additional funding to meet any new staffing requirements associated with our recommendation that CMS set an expectation for states to have a supervisory review program.

However, AHFSA noted what it considered to be conflicting assertions within the report. For example, it noted that we cited inexperienced staff as a factor that contributes to understatement but also appeared to take issue with the practice of supervisors changing reports prepared by inexperienced staff. While our report identifies a wide variety of factors that may contribute to understatement, we did not and could not meaningfully prioritize among these factors based on the responses of nursing home surveyors and state agency directors. We did find that many states were attempting to accomplish their survey workload with a large share of inexperienced surveyors and that state agency directors sometimes linked this reliance on inexperienced staff to the understatement of nursing home deficiencies. In addition, we found that frequent changes made during supervisory review were symptomatic of workforce shortages and survey methodology weaknesses. For example, surveyors who reported that survey teams had too many new surveyors, more often also reported either frequent changes to or removals of deficiencies during supervisory reviews. We believe that state quality assurance processes have the potential to play an important role in preventing understatement, which may result in states with inexperienced workforces relying more heavily on supervisory reviews.

AHFSA also stated that our report did not address limitations of federal monitoring surveys, specifically the potential inconsistency among CMS regional offices in how these surveys are conducted. Assessing CMS's performance on federal monitoring surveys was beyond the scope of this chapter. However, our May 2008 report noted several improvements CMS had made since fiscal years 2002 and 2003 in federal comparative surveys intended to make them more comparable to the state surveys they are assessing; these improvement include; (1) reducing the time between the state and federal surveys to ensure that they more accurately capture the conditions at the time of the state survey, (2) including at least half of the residents from state survey investigative samples to allow for a more clear- cut determination of whether the state survey should have cited a deficiency, and (3) using the same number of federal surveyors as the corresponding state survey, again to more closely mirror the conditions under which the state survey was conducted.[71]

Finally, AHFSA questioned whether the information that we received from surveyors about the IDR process was universally valid because their input about quality assurance reviews might be biased. Our methodology did not rely solely on surveyor responses to our questionnaire but used a separate questionnaire sent to state survey agency directors to help corroborate their responses. Thus we reported both that (1) over 40 percent of surveyors in four states indicated that their IDR process favored nursing home operators and (2) one state survey agency director agreed and three others acknowledged that frequent IDR hearings sometimes contributed to the understatement of deficiencies. We also collected and reported data on the number of deficiencies modified or overturned, which AHFSA said was a more accurate measure of the effect of IDRs.

We also incorporated technical comments from AHFSA as appropriate.

John E. Dicken
Director, Health Care

Appendix I: Scope and Methodology

This appendix describes the data and methods we used to identify the factors that contribute to the understatement of serious deficiencies on nursing home surveys.[72] This chapter relies largely on the data collected through (1) two GAO-administered Web-based questionnaires to nursing home surveyors and state agency directors and (2) analysis of federal and state nursing home survey results as reported in the federal monitoring survey database and the On-Line Survey, Certification, and Reporting (OSCAR) system. Summary results from the GAO questionnaires are available as an e-supplement to this chapter. See *Nursing Homes: Responses from Two Web-Based Questionnaires to Nursing Home Surveyors and State Agency Directors* (GAO-10-74SP), an E-supplement to GAO-10-70. To augment our quantitative analysis, we also interviewed officials at the Centers for Medicare & Medicaid (CMS) Survey and Certification Group and select regional offices;[73] reviewed federal regulations, guidance, and our prior work; and conducted follow-up interviews with eight state agency directors and a select group of surveyors. Except where otherwise noted, we used data from fiscal year 2007 because they were the most recently available data at the time of our analysis.

Development of Questionnaires and Analysis of Responses

We developed two Web-based questionnaires—one for the nursing home surveyors and one for the state agency directors.

Development of the Questionnaires

The questionnaires were developed and the data collection and analysis conducted to (1) minimize errors arising from differences in how a particular question might be interpreted and in the sources of informationavailable to respondents and (2) reduce variability in responses that should be qualitatively the same. GAO social science survey specialists aided in the design and development of both questionnaires. We pretestedthe two questionnaires with six surveyors from a local state and five former or current state agency directors, respectively. Based on feedback from these pretests, the questionnaires were revised to improve clarity and the precision of responses, and ensure that all questions were fair and unbiased. Most questions were closed-ended, which limited the respondent to answers such as yes or no, or to identifying the frequency that an event occurred using a scale—always, frequently, sometimes, infrequently, or never. For reporting purposes, we grouped the scaled responses into three categories—always/frequently, sometimes, and infrequently/never. Both questionnaires included some open-ended questions to allow respondents to identify specific training needs or other concerns.

With few exceptions, respondents entered their responses directly into the Web-based questionnaire databases.[74] These questionnaires were sent to the eligible population of nursing home surveyors and all state agency directors. We performed computer analyses to identify illogical or inconsistent responses and other indications of possible error. We also conducted follow-up interviews with select respondents to clarify and gain a contextual understanding of their responses.[75]

Questionnaire for Nursing Home Surveyors

This questionnaire was designed to gather information from nursing home surveyors nationwide about the process for identifying and citing nursing home deficiencies. It included questions about various aspects of the survey process identified by our prior work that may contribute to survey inconsistency and the understatement of deficiencies. Such aspects included survey methodology and guidance, deficiency determination, surveyor training, supervisory review of draft surveys, and state agency policies and procedures.[76]

We fielded the questionnaire from May through July 2008 to 3,819 eligible nursing home surveyors. To identify the eligible population, we downloaded a list of identification numbers for surveyors who had conducted at least one health survey of a nursing home in fiscal years 2006 or 2007 from CMS's OSCAR database and we obtained surveyors' e-mail addresses from state survey agencies. We received complete responses from 2,340 state surveyors, for a 61 percent response rate.[77] The state-level response rates were above 40 percent for all but three states— Connecticut, Illinois, and Pennsylvania.[78] We excluded Pennsylvania from our analysis because Pennsylvania's Deputy Secretary for Quality Assurance instructed the state's surveyors not to respond to our survey and few responded. (For response rates by state, see table 9.)

Table 9. Response Rates to GAO's Questionnaire of Nursing Home Surveyors, 2008

State	Number of respondents	Number of eligible surveyors	Response rate (in percent)
Alabama	36	52	69
Alaska	4	6	67
Arizona	19	28	68
Arkansas	28	54	52
California	306	544	56
Colorado	16	38	42
Connecticut	17	61	28
Delaware	13	16	81
District of Columbia	6	10	60
Florida	128	226	57
Georgia	47	54	87
Hawaii	4	7	57
Idaho	6	11	55
Illinois	34	171	20
Indiana	92	101	91
Iowa	37	59	63

Table 9 (Continued)			
Kansas	34	59	58
Kentucky	44	86	51
Louisiana	79	134	59
Maine	24	28	86
Maryland	29	47	62
Massachusetts	39	88	44
Michigan	50	80	63
Minnesota	58	85	68
Mississippi	21	35	60
State	**Number of respondents**	**Number of eligible surveyors**	**Response rate (in percent)**
Missouri	175	192	91
Montana	20	21	95
Nebraska	26	33	79
Nevada	21	25	84
New Hampshire	9	15	60
New Jersey	35	77	45
New Mexico	18	25	72
New York	108	250	43
North Carolina	53	84	63
North Dakota	12	16	75
Ohio	77	145	53
Oklahoma	63	92	68
Oregon	31	45	69
Rhode Island	20	27	74
South Carolina	15	27	56
South Dakota	20	22	91
Tennessee	52	79	66
Texas	201	281	72
Utah	16	25	64
Vermont	11	16	69
Virginia	36	42	86
Washington	60	85	71
West Virginia	14	22	64
Wisconsin	66	83	80
Wyoming	10	10	100.0
Total	**2,340**	**3,819**	**61**

Source: GAO.

Questionnaire for State Agency Directors

The questionnaire for state agency directors was designed to gather information on the nursing home survey process in each state. Directors were asked many of the same questions as the surveyors, but the survey agency directors' questionnaire contained additional questions on the overall organization of the survey agency, resource and staffing issues, CMS's Quality Indicator Survey (QIS), and experience with CMS's federal monitoring surveys.[79] In addition, the questionnaire for state agency directors asked them to rank the degree to which several factors, derived from our previous work, contributed to understatement.[80] This questionnaire was fielded from September to November 2008 to all 50 state survey agency directors and the survey agency director for the District of Columbia. We received completed responses from 50 of 51 survey agency directors, for a 98 percent response rate. The District of Columbia survey agency director did not respond.

Analysis of Responses

To analyze results from the survey questions among groups, we used standard descriptive statistics. In addition, we looked for associations between questions through correlations and tests of the differences in means for groups. For certain open-ended questions, we used a standard content review method to identify topics that respondents mentioned such as "applying CMS guidance," "on-the-job training," "time to complete survey onsite," or "time to complete the survey paperwork." Our coding process involved one independent coder and an independent analyst who verified a random sample of the coded comments. For open-ended questions that enabled respondents to provide additional general information, we used similar standard content review methods, including independent coding by two raters who resolved all disagreements through discussion.

Validity and Reliability of Data

In addition to the precautions taken during the development of the questionnaires, we performed automated checks on these data to identify inappropriate answers. We also reviewed the data for missing or ambiguous responses.[81] Where comments on open-ended questions provided more detail or contradicted responses to categorical questions, the latter were corrected. On the basis of the strength of our systematic survey processes and follow-up procedures, we determined that the questionnaire responses were representative of the experience and perceptions of nursing home surveyors and state agency directors nationally and at the state level, with the exception of Pennsylvania surveyors and the survey agency director of the District of Columbia. On the basis of the response rates and these activities, we determined that the data were sufficiently reliable for our purposes.

We also interviewed directors and other state agency officials in eight states to better understand unusual or interesting circumstances related to surveyor workforce and training, supervisory review, or state policies and practices. We selected these eight states based on our analysis of questionnaire responses from state agency directors and nursing home surveyors.

Analysis of Federal Comparative and Observational Surveys

We used information from our May 2008 report on federal comparative surveys nationwide for fiscal years 2002 through 2007 to categorize states into groups.[82] We used these results to identify states with high and low percentages of serious missed deficiencies.[83] We classified nine states as high-understatement states—those that had 25 percent or more federal comparative surveys identifying at least one missed deficiency at the actual harm or immediate jeopardy levels across all years. These states were Alabama, Arizona, Missouri, New Mexico, Oklahoma, South Carolina, South Dakota, Tennessee, and Wyoming. Zero-understatement states were those that had no federal comparative surveys identifying missed deficiencies at the actual harm or immediate jeopardy levels. These seven states were Alaska, Idaho, Maine, North Dakota, Oregon, Vermont, and West Virginia. Low-understatement states were the 10 with the lowest percentage of missed serious deficiencies (less than 6 percent)—Arkansas, Nebraska, Ohio, and all seven zero-understatement states.

Response rates among the high-, low-, and zero-understatement states— approximately 77, 62, and 71 percent, respectively—supported statistical testing of associations and differences among these state groupings. Therefore, in addition to descriptive statistics, we used correlations and tests of the differences in means for groups to identify questionnaire responses that were associated with differences in understatement.[84] We reported the statistically significant results for tests of association and differences between group averages at the 5 percent level, unless otherwise noted.

In a previous report, we found a possible relationship between the understatement of nursing home deficiencies on the federal comparative surveys and surveyor performance in General Investigation and Deficiency Determination on federal observational surveys—that is, high- understatement states more often had below-satisfactory ratings in General Investigation and Deficiency Determination than low- understatement states.[85] For this chapter, we applied the same statistical analysis to identify when responses to our questionnaires were associated with satisfactory performance on General Investigative and Deficiency Determination skills on the federal observational surveys. We interpreted such relationships as an indication of additional training needs.

Analysis of OSCAR

Analysis of OSCAR We used information from OSCAR and the federal monitoring survey databases to (1) compare the deficiencies cited by state and federal surveyors, (2) analyze the timing of nursing home surveys, and (3) assess trends in deficiency citations. OSCAR is a comprehensive database that contains information on the results of state nursing home surveys. CMS reviews these data and uses them to compute nursing home facility and state performance measures. When we analyzed these data, we included automated checks of data fields to ensure that they contain complete information. For these reasons, we determined that the OSCAR data were sufficiently reliable for our purposes.

- We used OSCAR and the federal monitoring survey database to compare average facility citations on state survey records with the average citations on federal observational survey records for the same facilities during fiscal years 2002 through 2007.[86] We computed the average number of serious deficiencies cited on federal observational surveys between fiscal years 2002 through 2007, and for the same facilities and time period, calculated the average number of serious deficiencies cited on state surveys. Next, we determined which facilities had greater average serious deficiency citations on federal observational surveys compared to state standard surveys between fiscal years 2002 through 2007. For these facilities, we computed the percentage difference between the average number of serious deficiencies cited on federal observational surveys and those cited on state surveys.
- We used OSCAR to determine the percentage of the most recent state surveys that were predictable because of their timing. Our analysis of survey predictability compared the time between state agencies' current and prior standard nursing home

surveys as of June 2008. According to CMS, states consider 9 months to 15 months from the last standard survey as the window for completing standard surveys because it yields a 12- month average. We considered surveys to be predictable if (1) homes were surveyed within 15 days of the 1-year anniversary of their prior survey or (2) homes were surveyed within 1 month of the maximum 15-month interval between standard surveys.

- We calculated the number of serious deficiencies on state surveys in OSCAR from calendar year 1999 through 2007. We examined the trend in G-level and higher deficiencies to assess whether CMS's expanded enforcement policy appeared to affect citation rates. Effective January 2000, CMS completed the implementation of its immediate-sanctions policy, requiring the referral of homes that caused actual harm or immediate jeopardy on successive standard surveys or intervening complaint investigations.

Appendix II: Comments from the Department of Health & Human Services

DEPARTMENT OF HEALTH & HUMAN SERVICES OFFICE OF THE SECRETARY

Assistant Secretary for Legislation
Washington, DC 20201

OCT 30 2009

John Dicken
Director, Health Care
U.S. Government Accountability Office
441 G Street N.W.
Washington, DC 20548

Dear Mr. Dicken:

Enclosed are comments on the U.S. Government Accountability Office's (GAO) report entitled: "NURSING HOMES: Addressing the Factors Underlying Understatement of Serious Care Problems Requires Sustained CMS and State Commitment" (GAO-10-70).

The Department appreciates the opportunity to review this report before its publication.

Sincerely,

Andrea Palm
Acting Assistant Secretary for Legislation

Enclosure

DEPARTMENT OF HEALTH & HUMAN SERVICES

Centers for Medicare & Medicaid Services

Administrator
Washington, DC 20201

DATE: OCT 30 2009

TO: Andrea Palm
Acting Assistant Secretary for Legislation
Office of the Secretary

FROM: Charlene Frizzera
Acting Administrator

SUBJECT: Government Accountability Office (GAO) Draft Report: "Nursing Homes: Addressing the Factors Underlying Understatement of Serious Care Problems Requires Sustained CMS and State Commitment" (GAO-10-70)

The Centers for Medicare & Medicaid Services (CMS) appreciates the opportunity to review and comment on the subject GAO Draft Report. The GAO was asked to examine four factors relevant to potential understatement of nursing home deficiencies including--

1. CMS' survey process;
2. Workforce shortages and training;
3. Supervisory reviews of surveys; and
4. State agency practices.

We believe that the GAO study adds value to the important public policy discussions regarding the survey process. The report derives its information primarily from opinion surveys of State surveyors and directors of State survey agencies. We particularly appreciate the GAO's effort to identify underlying causes of issues in the survey process and contribute ideas for solutions. We fully endorse five of the seven GAO recommendations. For the remaining two, we will convene a workgroup of State and Federal officials to explore alternate solutions that may be responsive to the intent of the GAO recommendations.

We offer the following, more detailed responses to the GAO recommendations.

GAO Recommendation 1: Quality Indicator Survey (QIS)

To improve the survey process, CMS must make sure measures are taken to address issues identified with the new QIS methodology.

Page 2 – Andrea Palm

CMS Response

We agree with this recommendation. We have designed the QIS specifically to improve consistency of survey processes and to provide both States and CMS with tools for continuous improvement. Since the tools for continuous improvement were not part of the original QIS design, their development has slowed QIS implementation somewhat, but the investment has been very worthwhile. A set of QIS "Desk Audit Reports" (DARs) represents one such tool. The DARs contain over 30 key investigative and decision-making factors for each QIS survey. The DARs also enable State survey supervisors to provide improved feedback to their surveyors, identify patterns in deficiency citation, and strengthen the consistency of the survey process between State surveyor teams. These tools provide information for the CMS regional offices and become part of a quarterly review teleconference in which each State can review the patterns of survey results together with the CMS regional office.

Finally, we established a user group that convenes quarterly to continue to address QIS issues as they arise. This user group may also represent a useful forum to share ideas for methods to facilitate implementation and to generate additional ideas for refinements to the system or to the implementation process. For example, Florida has just completed its statewide conversion from the traditional survey to the QIS and made a total revision to their surveyor orientation program materials. We plan to share these materials with the other States, so they can upgrade their orientation efforts to more effectively address the investigation and deficiency determination skills of newly hired surveyors.

GAO Recommendation 2: CMS Guidance for Surveyors

To improve guidance to surveyors, CMS should clarify and revise existing CMS written guidance to make it more concise, simplify its application in the field, and reduce confusion, particularly on the definition of actual harm.

CMS Response

We will seek alternate methods to address these issues, and will work with a workgroup of State and Federal officials to do so. We agree that it is desirable to clarify any areas of Federal guidance that may be ambiguous, but do not agree that shortening the guidance is necessarily the preferable method of doing so, or that greater conciseness would have the desired effect. One method of striking a balance between full guidance and conciseness may be to create some short reference documents for use in the field that contain cross-links back to the full guidance.

Based on previous GAO recommendations to ensure consistency, CMS embarked on a multi-year project to upgrade and clarify our interpretive guidelines for key regulations (Tags) in order to provide surveyors with accurate and up-to-date information in each topic area (such as nutrition, infection control, and incontinence, etc.). The guidance was developed with assistance from expert panels and is much more informative than previous guidance. We believe it is imperative for all surveyors to master the guidance and that the GAO's recommendation to bolster training efforts (recommendation #4) is the superior method, rather than seeking to shorten the guidance.

Many survey agencies that the revised guidance has enhanced the ability of their surveyors to correctly investigate concerns and select the correct levels of severity for non-compliance, including making distinctions as to when "actual harm" (Level 3) is reached for common types of deficient practices that fall under the various Tag topics. An example of a positive impact from revised guidance (in addressing deficiency understatement issues) can be seen in CMS' issuance of improved pharmacy guidelines. The new guidance clearly improved surveyors' ability to identify the use of unnecessary medications. Widely publicized concerns about the use of unnecessary medications had previously failed to alter the extent to which such problems were identified by surveyors. CMS issued the expanded guidance in late 2006 and combined the issuance with national training of surveyors. The percent of standard surveys in which unnecessary medications was identified by surveyors subsequently increased from the previously consistent rate of 13-14 percent in fiscal year (FY) 2000 through 2006 to 18 percent in FY 2007. These results are portrayed in Figure 1.

Fig. 1: Percent of Surveys Citing Unnecessary Drug Use

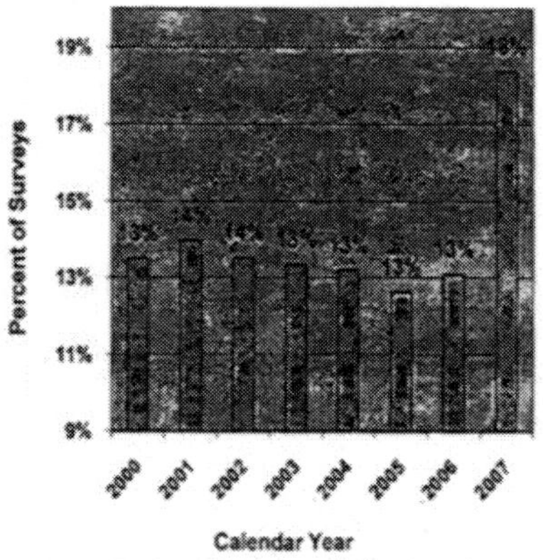

GAO Recommendation 3: Establish a National Pool of Surveyors for States

To address surveyor workforce shortages, CMS should consider establishing a pool of additional national surveyors that could augment State survey teams experiencing workforce shortages.

CMS Response

We do not plan to implement this recommendation, at least on any scale that would make a national difference. Section 1864 of the Social Security Act (the Act) directs the Secretary of the Department of Health and Human Services to enter into agreement with any State that is willing and capable of carrying out certain survey and certification responsibilities identified in the Act. According to the 1864 Agreement, the responsibility for conducting inspections and making recommendations for enforcement rests with the State survey agency. Establishing national survey teams to augment State surveys is problematic for a variety of reasons. First, it begins to blur the lines between (a) holding States accountable for meeting performance expectations versus (b) compensating for problematic performance due to State management decisions. While it is proper for CMS to set survey performance expectations and to establish qualifications for surveyor knowledge and training, we believe it is improper to tell States how to make personnel decisions, establish pay scales, recruit staff or, hire staff, or for CMS to try to alleviate State performance problems that arise because of State personnel management decisions. It is incumbent upon each State to determine alternate methods to fulfill the terms of the 1864 Agreement; it is not up to CMS to compensate for those State decisions.

Page 4 – Andrea Palm

While we have national contractors for some provider types (such as organ transplant centers and psychiatric hospitals), the use of national contractors has generally been limited to areas of specialty knowledge. The number of providers in many States may be so small that it is more cost-effective to have a national contractor than to contract with States and seek to maintain specialty surveyors for infrequent surveys. In those instances, we have offered the contracting to States and utilized a national contractor where States declined the offer. However, we regard as questionable the significant expansion of the use of national contractors to perform the more frequent nursing home surveys, in order to compensate for State performance issues.

We will explore this issue with our State-Federal workgroup in more detail in order to identify any circumstances in which a national pool may be advisable, and to identify any additional solutions. In the past, CMS has examined several promising practices with States and published policy briefs to assist States on issues such as surveyor recruitment strategies, retaining surveyors, and strategies to promote consistent surveyor performance.

GAO Recommendation 4: Training of Surveyors

To address insufficient training, CMS should (a) evaluate the current training programs and division of responsibility between Federal and State components to determine the most cost-effective approach; and (b) support the continuing education of experienced surveyors.

CMS Response

We agree with this recommendation. Training is critically important in fulfilling the mission of the survey and certification program. We have made significant investments to increase: (a) the number and types of CMS surveyor training courses, (b) the use of distance learning (satellites and Web-based training), and (c) the accessibility of training in geographical areas with large numbers of surveyors ("magnet areas").

Figure 2: Percent State Training Coordinators Not Satisfied with the Number of CMS Training Courses

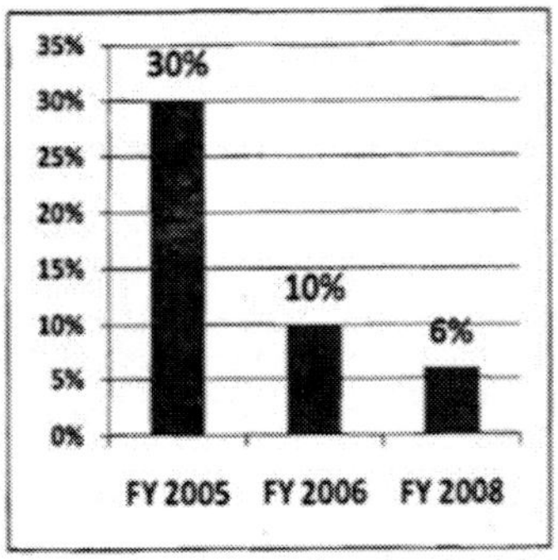

To increase the accessibility of training, we successfully inaugurated "Magnet Area Training (MAT)" in Florida and California. Evaluations of the training showed that MAT instruction produced results comparable to our other training events. We also initiated Web-based training (WBT) for one course in FY 2008, and we continue to develop new training courses that employ Web technology. These efforts have improved the survey and certification training profile. Figure 2, for example, shows the results of our annual survey of State training coordinators. The percent of respondents who indicated they were not satisfied with the number of CMS training courses declined from 30 percent in FY 2005 to 6 percent in FY 2008. The percent of respondents indicating they were satisfied increased from 30 percent in FY2005 to 41 percent in FY 2008.

Page 5 – Andrea Palm

While the trendline is very positive, the FY 2008 results still left 53 percent of participants indicating that they were only "somewhat satisfied." Gaps remain in both the number and types of courses.

As part of our ongoing dialogue with States, we will (a) poll States to complete a needs assessment for the continuing education of experienced surveyors; (b) offer selected continuing education opportunities based on the needs assessment; and (c) continue to expand the above initiatives.

GAO Recommendation 5: State Supervisory Reviews

To address inconsistencies in State supervisory reviews, CMS should set an expectation through guidance that States have a supervisory review program as a part of their Quality Assurance processes that includes routine reviews of deficiencies at the level of potential for more than minimal harm (D-F) and that provides feedback to surveyors regarding changes made to citations.

CMS Response

We agree with the recommendation. We will start by working with a State-Federal workgroup to identify promising practices, and initiate the process of setting more defined expectations for quality review. Historically, CMS has set forth expectations for documentation and for quality of the surveys, however, ensuring that deficiency determination and severity selection are consistent and accurate has been left to State management. We believe many States have developed effective programs or methods of supervisory review. Such methods include offsite review of citations and/or at least occasional participation onsite of a supervisor during deficiency decision-making meetings of surveyors, in order to coach and correct mistaken processes used by survey teams. In addition, CMS regional offices conduct validation reviews of State surveys and, particularly through the follow-along surveys, provide feedback to the State survey teams. We will build on these existing processes and identify additional steps that will be taken.

GAO Recommendation 6: Guidance on Non-Citation Practices

To address State agency practices and external pressure, CMS should reestablish expectations through guidance to State survey agencies that non-citation practices—official or unofficial—are inappropriate and systematically monitor trends in States' citations.

CMS Response

We agree with this recommendation. We will issue a Survey and Certification policy letter outlining our expectations regarding the survey and certification program as well as avenues to pursue if inappropriate practices are applied.

GAO Recommendation 7: Guidance on Communicating with CMS when External Pressures Exist

To address State agency practices and external pressure, CMS should establish expectations through guidance to State survey agencies to communicate and collaborate with their CMS Regional offices when they experience significant pressure from legislators or the nursing home industry that may have an impact on the survey process or surveyors' perceptions.

CMS Response

Page 6 – Andrea Palm

We agree with this recommendation. We will provide guidance for communicating surveyor concerns and provide feedback to State surveyors outlining our expectations regarding the survey and certification program, including avenues to pursue if inappropriate pressures are applied.

We appreciate the effort that went into this report and look forward to working with the GAO on this and other issues.

Related GAO Products

Nursing Homes: Opportunities Exist to Facilitate the Use of the Temporary Management Sanction. GAO-10-37R. Washington, D.C.: November 20, 2009.

Nursing Homes: CMS's Special Focus Facility Methodology Should Better Target the Most Poorly Performing Homes, Which Tended to Be Chain Affiliated and For-Profit. GAO-09-689. Washington, D.C.: August 28, 2009.

Medicare and Medicaid Participating Facilities: CMS Needs to Reexamine Its Approach for Funding State Oversight of Health Care Facilities. GAO-09-64. Washington, D.C.: February 13, 2009.

Nursing Homes: Federal Monitoring Surveys Demonstrate Continued Understatement of Serious Care Problems and CMS Oversight Weaknesses. GAO-08-517. Washington, D.C.: May 9, 2008.

Nursing Home Reform: Continued Attention Is Needed to Improve Quality of Care in Small but Significant Share of Homes. GAO-07-794T. Washington, D.C.: May 2, 2007.

Nursing Homes: Efforts to Strengthen Federal Enforcement Have Not Deterred Some Homes from Repeatedly Harming Residents. GAO-07-241. Washington, D.C.: March 26, 2007.

Nursing Homes: Despite Increased Oversight, Challenges Remain in Ensuring High-Quality Care and Resident Safety. GAO-06-117. Washington, D.C.: December 28, 2005.

Nursing Home Quality: Prevalence of Serious Problems, While Declining, Reinforces Importance of Enhanced Oversight. GAO-03-561. Washington, D.C.: July 15, 2003.

Nursing Homes: Quality of Care More Related to Staffing than Spending. GAO-02-431R. Washington, D.C.: June 13, 2002.

Nursing Homes: Sustained Efforts Are Essential to Realize Potential of the Quality Initiatives. GAO/HEHS-00-197. Washington, D.C.: September 28, 2000.

Nursing Home Care: Enhanced HCFA Oversight of State Programs Would Better Ensure Quality. GAO/HEHS-00-6. Washington, D.C.: November 4, 1999.

Nursing Homes: Proposal to Enhance Oversight of Poorly Performing Homes Has Merit. GAO/HEHS-99-157. Washington, D.C.: June 30, 1999.

Nursing Homes: Additional Steps Needed to Strengthen Enforcement of Federal Quality Standards. GAO/HEHS-99-46. Washington, D.C.: March 18, 1999.

California Nursing Homes: Care Problems Persist Despite Federal and State Oversight. GAO/HEHS-98-202. Washington, D.C.: July 27, 1998.

End Notes

[1] Medicare is the federal health care program for elderly and certain disabled individuals. Medicaid is a joint federal-state health care financing program for certain categories of low- income individuals.

[2] In addition to the oversight of nursing homes, CMS and state survey agencies are responsible for oversight of other Medicare and Medicaid providers, such as home health agencies, intermediate care facilities for the mentally retarded, and hospitals.

[3] See a list of related GAO products at the end of this chapter.

[4] See GAO, *Nursing Homes: Federal Monitoring Surveys Demonstrate Continued Understatement of Serious Care Problems and CMS Oversight Weaknesses*, GAO-08-517 (Washington, D.C.: May 9, 2008).

[5] CMS's Survey and Certification Group is responsible for ensuring the effectiveness of state survey activities and managing the federal monitoring survey program.

[6] See GAO, *Nursing Home Quality: Prevalence of Serious Problems, While Declining, Reinforces Importance of Enhanced Oversight*, GAO-03-561 (Washington, D.C.: July 15, 2003) and GAO, *Nursing Home Reform: Continued Attention Is Needed to Improve Quality of Care in Small but Significant Share of Homes*, GAO-07-794T (Washington, D.C.: May 2, 2007). In response to our recommendation to finalize the development, testing, and implementation of a more rigorous survey methodology, CMS evaluated and is currently implementing a revised survey methodology.

[7] See GAO, *Nursing Homes: Despite Increased Oversight, Challenges Remain in Ensuring High-Quality Care and Resident Safety*, GAO-06-117 (Washington, D.C.: Dec. 28, 2005).

[8] See GAO-03-561. Our analysis of survey predictability considered surveys to be predictable if (1) homes were surveyed within 15 days of the 1-year anniversary of the prior survey or (2) homes were surveyed within 1 month of the maximum 15-month interval between standard surveys. We used this rationale because homes know the maximum allowable interval between surveys, and those whose prior surveys were conducted 14 or 15 months earlier are aware that they are likely to be surveyed soon.

[9] See GAO-03-561.

[10] See GAO-03-561.

[11] Eligible surveyors are those who had conducted at least one health survey of a nursing home in fiscal year 2006 or 2007 and for whom we could obtain an e-mail or other address from their state survey agency.

[12] We excluded Pennsylvania from our analysis because Pennsylvania's Deputy Secretary for Quality Assurance instructed the state's surveyors not to respond to our survey. Two other states had response rates below 40 percent—Connecticut (28 percent), and Illinois (20 percent). Illinois' response rate probably reflected that surveyors' access to their e-mail accounts and our Web-based survey was limited to only 1 day per month.

[13] The District of Columbia agency director did not respond to our questionnaire.

[14] We did not ask nursing home surveyors a similar question because survey agency directors, as a result of their positions, were a more consistent source of knowledge about the influence of these factors on understatement.

[15] See GAO-08-517. This database captures the results of two types of federal monitoring surveys. Federal comparative surveys are conducted independently by federal surveyors to evaluate state surveys. Federal surveyors resurvey a home that was recently inspected by state surveyors and compare the deficiencies identified during the two surveys. When federal surveyors accompany state surveyors to directly observe them during a nursing home survey it is considered a federal observational survey.

[16] We use the term survey record to refer to CMS's Form 2567, which is the official statement of deficiencies with respect to federal quality standards.

[17] Other areas include Admission, Transfer and Discharge Rights, Resident Rights, Resident Behavior and Facility Practices, Nursing Services, Pharmacy Services, Dietary Services, Physician Services, Specialized Rehabilitative Services, Dental Services, Infection Control, and Physical Environment. Surveys also examine compliance with federal fire safety requirements.

[18] Revisits are not required for most deficiencies cited below the actual-harm level—that is, A through F.

[19] Nursing homes can also appeal deficiency citations, which result in hearings before an administrative law judge; nursing homes may also request HHS's Departmental Appeals Board to review.

[20] On-site sources include observations, interviews, and records review.

[21] See GAO-03-561.

[22] The federal government funds state surveys through the Medicare and Medicaid programs. States contribute a share of Medicaid and non-Medicaid funds to support survey activities. State non-Medicaid contributions are to reflect the benefit states derive from health care facilities that meet federal quality standards as well as the cost of assessing compliance with state licensing requirements. See GAO, *Medicare and Medicaid Participating Facilities: CMS Needs to Reexamine Its Approach for Funding State Oversight of Health Care Facilities*, GAO-09-64 (Washington, D.C.: Feb. 13, 2009).

[23] See GAO-09-64.

[24] See GAO-03-561.

[25] CMS commented on the importance of quality-assurance processes and noted it had already incorporated such reviews into CMS regional offices' reviews of the state performance standards. However, the agency did not require states to initiate an ongoing process that would evaluate the appropriateness of the scope and severity of documented deficiencies, as we recommended. See GAO-03-561.

[26] See GAO-03-561.

[27] In addition to the federal monitoring surveys, CMS established annual state performance reviews in fiscal year 2001 to measure a state's compliance with specific standards. These standards generally focus on the timeliness and quality of surveys, complaint investigations, and enforcement actions. CMS's state performance reviews include (1) an examination of the quality of state survey agency investigations and decision making and (2) the timeliness and quality of complaint investigations.

[28] In 1998, the Health Care Financing Administration, the HHS agency now known as CMS, acknowledged the need to perform a greater number of comparative surveys and have done so. Between October 1998 and July 1999 only about 9 percent (64) of federal monitoring surveys were comparative. However, in our May 2008 report, we found that for the period of fiscal years 2002 through 2007 about 20 percent (976) of federal monitoring surveys were comparative surveys and the remaining 80 percent were observational surveys. By statute, comparative surveys must be conducted within 2 months of the completion of the state survey.

[29] CMS began requiring regional offices to make this determination in fiscal year, 2002 and it is captured by a yes/no validation question.

[30] See GAO-08-517.

[31] In May 2008, we found that understatement also occurred when state survey teams cited deficiencies at too low a level of scope and severity. At that time, CMS did not require federal surveyors to evaluate scope and severity differences between state and federal comparative surveys. However, as of October 2008, CMS began requiring such assessments.

[32] See GAO-08-517.

[33] For purposes of this chapter, we defined the federal nursing home survey process as both the traditional methodology used to evaluate compliance of nursing homes with federal requirements and the written guidance provided by CMS to help state agencies carry out survey activities.

[34] Survey methodology is defined as the traditional approach used to evaluate nursing home compliance with federal regulations as outlined by CMS in Appendix P of the SOM.

[35] For purposes of this chapter, we defined CMS written guidance as the information in the SOM on the long-term care survey process, including the survey protocol for long-term care facilities in Appendix P and the guidance on federal quality standards in Appendix PP as well as any additional materials provided by CMS to assist surveyors, such as Survey and Certification letters.

[36] Guidance for determining actual–harm level deficiencies is provided in Section IV, Appendix P of the SOM.

[37] See GAO-03-561.

[38] Federal nursing home quality standards detail requirements for the delivery of care, resident outcomes, and facility conditions. State survey teams use these federal quality standards to assess compliance during state nursing home surveys.

[39] In October 2000, CMS began revising investigative protocols for assessing specific deficiencies. The intent of this initiative is to enable surveyors to better (1) identify specific deficiencies, (2) investigate whether a deficiency is the result of poor care, and (3) document the level of harm resulting from a home's identified deficient care practices. See GAO-03-561.

[40] Our questionnaire included 13 topics of the approximately 200 federal quality standards. Seven of these were taken from the Quality of Care category of federal quality standards, the others originated from different categories such as Resident Assessment and Dietary Services. See GAO-08-517.

[41] Beginning January 1, 1999, CMS directed states to avoid scheduling surveys for the same month of the year as a nursing home's previous survey. However, surveys can also be considered predictable if occurring at a time other than near the 1-year anniversary or 15-month maximum date. For example, nursing home operators could be alerted when the state agency is surveying a facility in a nearby area if all the facilities in that area were surveyed at about the same time.

[42] In 2003, we found that 34 percent of nursing home surveys were predictable. See GAO-03-561.

[43] According to CMS, states consider 9 months to 15 months from the last standard survey as the window for completing standard surveys because it yields a 12-month average. Thus, to maintain an average survey interval of 12 months, given that some facilities are not surveyed until near or after 15 months, more surveys would need to occur within 9 months of the last standard survey. See GAO-06-117.

[44] At the time of our survey, the QIS methodology was being implemented in eight state agencies: Connecticut, Florida, Kansas, Louisiana, Minnesota, New Mexico, North Carolina, and Ohio. According to a CMS official, Connecticut is the only one of these states that has implemented the QIS statewide. As of May 2008, CMS projected that the QIS would be fully implemented in all states in 2014.

[45] The QIS evaluation was conducted to answer questions about accuracy, documentation, changes in the number and types of deficiencies, and whether the QIS process is more efficient. HHS, CMS, *Evaluation of the Quality Indicator Survey (QIS), Final Report* (December 2007), http//:www.cms.hhs.gov/CertificationandComplianc/ Downloads/ QISExecSummary.pdf (accessed July 17, 2009).

[46] Scope refers to the number of residents potentially or actually affected and has three levels—isolated, pattern, and widespread. A pattern scope refers to deficiencies at the B, E, H, and K levels and a widespread scope refers to deficiencies at the C, F, I, and L levels.

[47] We asked all 42 directors who had not participated in the QIS to provide their opinions on the new methodology; we received comments from 18 of the 42 directors.

[48] See GAO-03-561.

[49] Virginia did not provide the information needed to compute a vacancy rate.

[50] Michigan and Illinois did not provide this information.

[51] See GAO-09-64.

[52] This information was last updated in June 2009 before the governor of California signed the state's budget revisions.

[53] Seven states did not report the number of surveyors with less than 2 years of experience—Illinois, Michigan, Minnesota, Texas, Washington, West Virginia, and Wisconsin.

[54] Revisit surveys are generally conducted in facilities when a G-level or higher deficiency is cited by a survey team, to verify that serious deficiencies have been corrected by the home.

[55] In an open-ended question at the end of the questionnaire, 842 surveyors commented on a wide range of topics related to surveys. These comments represented about 36 percent of all nursing home surveyor respondents; 15 percent of the comments represented about 6 percent of all respondents.

[56] The 476 surveyors who responded to this open-ended question about training needs constituted about 20 percent of all respondents.

[57] For supervisory review processes, we defined direct-line supervisors as including survey team leaders, direct supervisors, and supervisors at district or regional offices. Central state agency staff was defined as including quality assurance teams, legal counsel, state training coordinators, and compliance specialists.

[58] These review steps could be done at the direct-line supervisor level or by central state agency staff. The difference between supervisory review levels for surveys with J through L citations and those for surveys with D through F citations was significant at the 1 percent level.

[59] Forty states review a sample of all draft surveys. Such reviews may include additional examination of surveys with deficiencies at either the D through F or J through L levels.

[60] See GA0-03-561.

[61] Seventy-four percent of state agency directors indicated that inadequate supervisory review processes infrequently or never contributed to understatement in their state, and 4 percent of state agency directors were unsure or had no opinion on this topic.

[62] CMS previously identified the existence of a potential noncitation practice in one state that had an unusually high number of homes with no deficiencies on their standard surveys. Contrary to federal guidance, surveyors in that state were not citing all identified deficiencies but rather brought them to the homes' attention with the expectation that the deficiencies would be corrected. See GAO-03-561.

[63] CMS requires on-site revisits for any noncompliance identified at level F (with a finding of substandard quality of care) or any level higher than F.

[64] Effective January 2000, CMS expanded its immediate sanctions policy, requiring referral of homes found to have harmed one or a small number of residents (G-level deficiencies) on successive routine surveys or intervening complaint investigations.

[65] CMS officials previously acknowledged that the double G policy may have had an unintended negative effect on the rate of deficiency citations. See GAO, *Nursing Homes: Efforts to Strengthen Federal Enforcement Have Not Deterred Some Homes from Repeatedly Harming Residents*, GAO-07-241 (Washington, D.C.: Mar. 26, 2007).

[66] In this section, we refer to two states we interviewed as State A and State B to maintain confidentiality for the officials from these state agencies. The corresponding regional offices are referred to as regional office responsible for State A or State B, respectively.

[67] Alaska, Hawaii, Illinois, and West Virginia did not report information on the number of IDRs.

[68] The following states did not report the number of deficiencies deleted or downgraded through the IDR process: Alaska, Hawaii, Illinois, Kentucky, Nebraska, New Jersey, New Mexico, Vermont, or West Virginia. Maine, Oklahoma, Utah, Washington, and Wyoming provided the number of deficiencies deleted but not the number that were downgraded.

[69] According to CMS guidance, if an outside entity conducts the IDR, the results of the process may serve only as a recommendation to the state survey agency of noncompliance or compliance with the federal requirements for nursing homes.

[70] See GAO-03-561.

[71] See GAO-08-517.

[72] This chapter follows and expands on our May 2008 report, which examined (1) the information contained in federal monitoring surveys about understatement nationwide, and (2) CMS management and oversight of the federal monitoring survey program, see GAO-08-517.

[73] CMS's Survey and Certification Group is responsible for ensuring the effectiveness of state survey activities and managing the federal monitoring survey program.

[74] We mailed paper copies of the questionnaire to 15 surveyors in Arkansas, who did not have a state-issued e-mail address; on request, an additional copy was faxed to a surveyor. Seven out of the 16 paper copies were completed and returned to GAO.

[75] Although nursing home surveyors' responses were anonymous to preserve their confidentiality, a few surveyors voluntarily provided their contact information and agreed to be interviewed.

[76] Questions about CMS's survey methodology directed surveyors to respond about the traditional survey methodology, not the new Quality Indicator Survey (QIS) methodology, which had been implemented in eight states.

[77] When respondents indicated that they did not conduct health safety surveys of nursing homes and therefore should have been excluded from the population of eligible nursing home surveyors, these surveyors and their responses were excluded.

[78] The Illinois response rate likely reflects that surveyors' access to their e-mail accounts, and our Web-based survey, was limited to only 1 day per month.

[79] All state agency directors were asked about CMS's traditional survey methodology, which all states used in 2008. However eight state agency directors, who indicated that the QIS has been implemented in at least part of their states, were asked additional questions specifically about the QIS.

[80] We did not ask nursing home surveyors a similar question because survey agency directors, as a result of their positions, were a more consistent source of knowledge about the influence of these factors on understatement.

[81] Where responses to particular questions were fewer than the overall number of responses for the questionnaire, this limitation is indicated in the text.

[82] During this period, fiscal year 2002 was the first year that the database contained all the information needed to assess the results of federal comparative surveys. (See GAO-08-517.)

[83] Federal comparative surveys are done on a small group of facilities that are not randomly selected, and the understatement of deficiencies identified through comparative surveys are not representative of all nursing home surveys or survey teams within each state.

[84] For our descriptive statistics, we computed means, the minimum and maximum responses, responses at the 25th, 50th, and 75th percentiles, frequencies among categories of respondents, such as those from high- and low-

understatement states, as well as frequencies across two or more categories of respondents. Correlations were computed as Pearson's correlations of association. T-tests were done to identify when the mean response from two different categories of respondents, such as high- and low-understatement states, were significantly different from each other.

[85] GAO-08-517. The General Investigation segment assesses the effectiveness of state survey team actions such as collection of information, discussion of survey observations, interviews with nursing home residents, and implementation of CMS investigative protocols. The Deficiency Determination segment evaluates the skill with which the state survey teams (1) integrate and analyze all information collected and (2) use the guidance for surveyors and identify deviations from regulatory requirements.

[86] We use the term survey record to refer to CMS's Form 2567, which is the official statement of deficiencies with respect to federal quality standards.

In: Nursing Homes Quality and Care Issues
Editor: Carlos E. Melendez
ISBN: 978-1-61668-855-4

Chapter 3

NURSING HOME TRANSPARENCY, ENFORCEMENT & QUALITY IMPROVEMENT HEARING*

Herb Kohl

Good Afternoon. I call this hearing to order, and welcome our witnesses. In May, this Committee held a hearing to examine the legacy of the 1987 Nursing Home Reform Act. We heard from various experts on just how far nursing homes have come in the past twenty years. While our previous hearing was about looking back, today's hearing is about moving forward and taking the next big step in improving our nation's nursing homes. To do so, I have been working with my colleague Senator Grassley on a proposal to improve nursing home quality by increasing transparency and strengthening enforcement. We are pleased to have Senator Grassley here to address the committee today.

We believe that Americans should have access to as much information about a nursing home as possible, including the results of government inspections, the number of staff employed at a home, and information about the home's ownership. The government should ensure that consumers can obtain this information in a clear, timely, and accurate manner so that they can make the right decision about where to place a loved one.

Our bill will also strengthen the government's system of enforcement. Under the current system, nursing homes that are not providing good care, or—even worse—are putting their residents in harms way, can escape penalty from the government while they slip in and out of compliance with federal regulations. This is unacceptable. We need the threat of sanctions to mean something—and under my bill with Senator Grassley, they will. We also need to make sure that regulators are able to intervene quickly in order to protect the safety of residents.

Today we will also hear from CMS Acting Administrator Kerry Weems. While working on our bill with CMS, we have discovered that many of our goals are aligned. Administrator Weems will testify shortly about the Special Focus Facility Program created by CMS to deal

* This is an edited, reformatted and augmented version of a U. S. Government Accountability Office publication dated November 15, 2007

with those nursing homes exhibiting a consistent history of providing poor care to residents. We will be asking him about a significant move toward transparency that CMS is planning to undertake. In just over two weeks, CMS will be disclosing the names of the facilities taking part in the Special Focus Facility Program.

I am pleased to say CMS is beating us to the punch: disclosing this list is a provision in our forthcoming bill. CMS understands what we understand—that it is in everybody's best interest to let consumers know which nursing homes repeatedly demonstrate deficiencies and violate government standards. Those homes are obviously not doing their jobs. Often the only way to ensure the improvement of any entity is to bring its failings to light. Senator Grassley feels that way, CMS feels that way, and I feel that way. I honestly believe that more nursing homes will come back into compliance for good if they have the court of public opinion and the power of market forces as encouragement.

At the same time, we acknowledge that our goal is not to close a home, but to fix the home, because that is often what is best for the residents. As you will hear, the Special Focus Facility Program is helping these facilities make the changes needed to improve care.

Our hearing today also features a third panel of distinguished witnesses. And in a rare stroke of good fortune, three of them come to us from Wisconsin! We will hear recommendations from national experts, organized labor, and representatives of the nursing home industry on the topics of transparency and enforcement.

As always, I find it very important to state that while we are shining a light on poor-performing homes, we believe that a vast majority of nursing homes are doing a good job. Most homes provide exemplary care—the type of care you would be happy to have a member of your own family receive. We will hear from one such home today, Marquardt Memorial Manor in Watertown, Wisconsin. I can vouch for this home personally, as I have the opportunity to visit many times.

Thank you all for being here. I look forward to working with you during the coming weeks as Senator Grassley and I complete our policy, and I welcome my colleagues on the Aging Committee to contribute their legislative ideas as well. We will now turn to Senator Grassley for his remarks.

In: Nursing Homes Quality and Care Issues
Editor: Carlos E. Melendez
ISBN: 978-1-61668-855-4

Chapter 4

NURSING HOME TRANSPARENCY, ENFORCEMENT & QUALITY IMPROVEMENT HEARING*

Steve Biondi

Thank you Chairman Kohl, Ranking Member Smith, and members of the Committee. I appreciate the opportunity to be here today representing the American Health Care Association (AHCA) and our profession's perspective on how to increase transparency, accountability, and meaningful information that can help consumers evaluate long term care quality as well as how we can continue to work together and toward our mutual objective of always providing optimal patient care.

My name is Steve Biondi, and I am Vice President for Clinical Services with Extendicare Health Services, based in Milwaukee, Wisconsin. I oversee regulatory compliance, which includes ensuring that Extendicare's 200 long term care facilities across North America achieve and maintain regulatory compliance. Extendicare employs 34,000 people and the capacity to care for nearly 27,000 patients and residents.

I am a registered nurse (RN), a licensed nursing home administrator (LNHA), and have worked as an ombudsman. I am certified as a surveyor by the Centers for Medicare & Medicaid Services (CMS) and have conducted national satellite education programs for surveyors on adult abuse prevention and survey, certification, and enforcement for CMS' precursor, the Health Care Financing Administration. Early on, I worked for the State of Florida's Department of Health and Rehabilitation Services and was appointed by then Governor Graham to oversee licensure and certification of nursing homes in South Florida, Medicaid approval and payment, pre-admission assessment, adult abuse investigation, and other programs where I was involved with revoking and decertifying three facilities due to inadequate quality outcomes.

As a member of the American Health Care Association (AHCA), I co-chair the Association's Survey/Regulatory Committee, which focuses on quality, federal survey,

---

* This is an edited, reformatted and augmented version of a U. S. Senate Special Committee on Aging publication dated November 16, 2007.

certification, enforcement, and regulatory issues related to quality. I serve concurrently on the Quality Improvement Committee, which seeks to advance the use of evidenced-based practices, and to build leadership competencies for AHCA membership.

I am proud to represent my fellow long term care providers and a profession that has embraced quality. We know that you, Mr. Chairman, and the members of this committee understand the myriad issues surrounding the long term care of some of our nation's most vulnerable citizens. We acknowledge your salutary commitment to ensuring our seniors receive the quality care they need and deserve – as evidenced by your leadership with this committee and introduction of legislation such as the *Patient Safety and Abuse Prevention Act of 2007 (S. 1577),* which AHCA supports.

I also wish to commend Senators Gordon Smith, Blanche Lincoln, and Susan Collins, who have put forward some of the most important regulatory reform concepts of the past twenty years – systematic reforms to the survey and certification process, and other critical changes that can help to build mutually beneficial partnerships, and undo an era of unproductive confrontation. The Smith-Lincoln-Collins *Long Term Care Quality and Modernization Act of 2007 (S. 1980)* represents an important step toward establishing more broadly such a culture of partnership – one we enthusiastically embrace and endorse.

Mr. Chairman, as today's hearing focuses on federal, state, and industry initiatives to improve nursing home transparency and survey and enforcement, along with the quality of services in the country's 16,000 nursing homes, I submit that part of the challenge before us is to work together – collaboratively – to promote transparency across the board.

By this, I mean expanding the concept of transparency beyond just facilities to include the survey and enforcement process itself. Doing so would enhance facilities' efforts to improve patient care, and would mirror our profession's own quality improvement initiatives. We believe that working together and creating a "culture of cooperation" is imperative—it is how we can continue to improve the quality of care and quality of life for the millions of patients (patients is used to refer to both long term care patients and residents) and families who rely on us everyday for the long term care and services they need.

Commitment to Quality

We have made tremendous strides in the twenty years since Congress enacted the *Omnibus Budget Reconciliation Act of 1987 (OBRA '87)*, which included the *Nursing Home Reform Act.* Earlier this year, as this Committee explored *OBRA's* history, its intent, and why it was a milestone piece of legislation, one factor that was undeniable twenty years ago, is undeniable today, and that will be undeniable twenty years from now is the unbreakable link between stable funding and quality.

That link has been recognized repeatedly by the Centers for Medicare & Medicaid Services, including in its recommendation that skilled nursing facilities receive a 3.3 percent Medicare market basket update for FY 2008 that states, "These new payment rates reflect our commitment to improving the quality of care in the long-term care setting while maintaining predictability and stability in payments for the nursing home industry...."

In an article written by then-Acting Administrator of CMS Leslie Norwalk for the May 2007 issue of *Provider* magazine, Ms. Norwalk observed:

> *Long before hospitals, doctors, home health providers, pharmacies, dialysis facilities and others came to the table, the nursing home industry was out front with Quality First – a volunteer effort to elevate quality and accountability.... Advancing Excellence in America's Nursing Homes... builds on the 2001 Quality First campaign and stresses the essential connection between quality, adequate payment for services and financial stability.*

Just as stable funding fosters quality, quality improvement centers on greater disclosure, transparency and accountability – all of which must be continued and expanded.

These central tenets of quality improvement initiatives represent the core of *Advancing Excellence in America's Nursing Homes. Advancing Excellence* is a coalition effort, co-founded by AHCA and comprised of providers, caregivers, researchers, government agencies, workers and consumers. The campaign builds on previous initiatives and focuses on specific, measurable quality improvement goals supported by evidence-based information and a national infrastructure. The campaign is designed to cultivate greater partnership both nationally and at the state level, which is ameliorating the sometimes adversarial atmosphere among these groups as they work together to ensure that patients in their communities receive the highest quality long term care.

Nearly 6,200 facilities – about 39 percent of nursing homes nationwide – are participating in the voluntary *Advancing Excellence* campaign, which AHCA continues to promote among our membership.

Nursing homes participating in the *Advancing Excellence* campaign select both clinical quality goals and organizational improvement goals to achieve consistent delivery of better quality care by enhancing staff performance. One of the hallmarks of the campaign is the evidence-based resources provided to nursing homes as well as access to support from the Quality Improvement Organizations (QIOs). The campaign culled best practices and other materials that give nursing home staff the information and tools needed to improve on clinical quality goals such as minimizing high and low risk pressure ulcers, ensuring patients remain independent to the best of their ability, minimizing pain experienced by longer-term patients and those patients admitted to nursing homes from hospital settings.

Measuring Quality Improvement

We are making progress and reporting on that progress. In fact, the clinical quality goals align with data tracked by CMS through the Online Survey, Certification and Reporting (OSCAR) system and publicly reported and posted to its *Nursing Home Compare* website.

OSCAR data clearly points to improvements in patient outcomes, increases in overall direct care staffing levels, and significant decreases in quality of care survey deficiencies. At the same time, an independent analysis confirms consistently high patient and family satisfaction with the care and services provided.

Specifically, the data shows:

- There is a positive trend in the quality measures posted on *Nursing Home Compare* with improvements in key areas for short-term and long stay patients in pain, restraints, and pressure ulcers.

- Pain for long term stay patients was vastly improved from a rate of 10.7 percent in 2002 to 4.6 percent in 2007.
- Pain in short-term patients was reduced from 25.4 percent in 2002 to 20.7 percent in 2007.
- Use of physical restraints for long stay patients dropped from 9.7 percent in 2002 to 5.6 percent in 2007.
- For short-term patients, the pressure ulcer measure also improved – from 20.4 percent in 2002 to 17.5 percent in 2007.

Assessing Patient & Family Satisfaction

In addition to improving clinical quality, we are evaluating consumer satisfaction and staffing as it relates to quality. A 2006 benchmark study, which included approximately 2,500 AHCA member facilities, indicated that a vast majority – more than four out of five – of nursing facilities have very high customer satisfaction ratings. In these 83 percent of facilities, patients and family members stated that they would recommend their facility – a clear indication of quality.

In May 2007, My InnerView, Inc. (MIV), which offers Web-based quality management systems, released its independent second annual report on patient and family satisfaction for the care and services provided in nursing facilities. For two consecutive years, more than four out of five of the more than 92,000 individuals indicated high overall satisfaction. The latest report indicates that 82 percent of the respondents would assess their overall satisfaction as good or excellent. Further, 88 percent of respondents rated the nursing care as either good or excellent.

Long Term Care Workforce

An essential element to providing quality care is having well-trained, qualified staff—that is why two of the organizational improvement goals for *Advancing Excellence* relate to staffing.

We already suffer from a nursing shortage, which is exacerbated by a nurse educator shortage. Nationally, more than 15 percent of registered nurse (RN), 13 percent of licensed practical nurse (LPN), and 8 percent of certified nursing aide (CNA) positions – nearly 100,000 vacancies overall – have been identified and the current long term caregiver shortage is only projected to get progressively worse over the next decade. So, attracting, training, and retaining quality long term care staff remains a particular challenge for long term care providers. AHCA has been working with the U.S. Department of Labor to address some of the critical issues regarding workforce, but clearly Congress has a critical role to play in ameliorating some of the workforce issues.

It is important to note one particular research study of the current Survey & Certification process and its impact on the long term care workforce. Long term care researcher, Vivian Tellis-Nayak, PhD, recently highlighted the fact that nursing home administrators are often discouraged by a survey process that seeks to identify faults, rather than to encourage quality.

Tellis-Nayak notes that the state survey "is confrontational and leaves no room for collaboration. It is uncaring and punitive, not educational." This view of the survey system is shared by many of the staff in nursing facilities nationwide. In order to address these shortfalls of the current system, we must move toward a "culture of cooperation" where stakeholders work in tandem to promote enhanced outcomes, rather than sensationalize shortcomings. *OBRA '87* took the first step in promoting care quality and standards of excellence for long term care – passage of the *Long Term Care Quality and Modernization Act of 2007* today can take us the next step.

SPECIAL FOCUS FACILITIES

AHCA has been working proactively with CMS for more than a year to address concerns with its Special Focus Facility Initiative. Recent revisions from the agency allow for notification of the State Medicaid Agency and the State Ombudsman Office when a facility is designated as a "Special Focus Facility." While AHCA is pleased that CMS accepted our recommendation to require that a facility's administrator, owners, and governing bodies also be notified should a facility be designated for "special focus," we are concerned about CMS' plan to make that designation public by adding a hyperlink to the *Nursing Home Compare* website. Adding such a notation on this public website is more likely to alarm patients, families, and health care consumers who have little background or understanding with respect to what it means to be a Special Focus Facility.

CMS has been slow to adopt any transparency around its Special Focus Facility Initiative. We remain concerned that CMS has not been forthcoming with details about the formula used to identify special focus facilities and the specific criteria a facility must meet to remove the special focus designation.

EXPANDING THE ROLE OF THE QUALITY IMPROVEMENT ORGANIZATIONS

The Quality Improvement Organizations (QIOs) play a vital role in long term care. The Agency for Healthcare Research and Quality's (AHRQ's) second annual *State Snapshots* based on the *National Healthcare Quality Report* highlights how – through an ongoing partnership and cooperation between the QIOs and individual nursing homes in every state – the QIOs are helping to improve quality in our nation's nursing homes.

All nursing homes in every state can access basic improvement assistance from their state QIO, and a subset of nursing homes in each state receive more intensive QIO assistance. Recent CMS data on nursing home performance strongly suggests that when QIOs partner with individual nursing homes, patient outcomes improve. Data collected between the fourth quarter of 2004 and the fourth quarter of 2006 shows that all nursing facilities across the country averaged a 9 percent relative improvement in the incidence of pressure ulcers and a 21 percent relative reduction in the use of physical restraints. But the facilities receiving intensive QIO assistance achieved a laudable 16 percent relative improvement in pressure ulcers and a 32 percent relative improvement in pain management.

Looking ahead, Mr. Chairman, we believe Medicare should fund an expanded role for QIOs in improving quality outcomes in all nursing homes and most importantly, those considered poor performers. According to a recent study from The Commonwealth Fund entitled, "Medicare's Quality Improvement Organization Program Value in Nursing Homes" published in the Spring 2007 *Health Care Financing Review*, which specifically looked at QIOs' work with nursing homes, suggests that "based on measurable improvements in residents' quality of life, the QIO program is a sound investment of health care dollars."

Accelerating efforts to strengthen and broaden the system of quality measurement in nursing homes, just as Medicare is doing in hospitals and physician office practices, will also lead to even greater improvement.

Stakeholder Collaboration to Address Poor Performing Facilities

In June, Mr. Chairman, AHCA and American Association of Homes and Services for the Aging (AAHSA) reached out to AARP, which convened a group of stakeholders, including the Long Term Care Ombudsman, National Citizens' Coalition for Nursing Home Reform (NCCNHR), and CMS to discuss "poor performing facilities," and to identify how we could intervene and help a facility improve, before being designated as a Special Focus Facility.

Subsequently, a subgroup tackled this issue and developed several recommendations that will be evaluated by the larger group of stakeholders and that we would be pleased to share with this committee sometime in 2008. Again, we are proud to be working collaboratively and cooperatively with other long term care stakeholders in addressing a problem requiring aggressive action.

Consumer-Friendly Resources

Clearly, family and ombudsmen involvement within facilities are key components to improving quality. AHCA has long encouraged family members to stay involved when a loved one is receiving care in a long term care facility. This year, AHCA acknowledged the extraordinary involvement of one such family member—Benjamin Thacker—who we recognized as "AHCA's Young Adult Volunteer of the Year." The 18-year old high school senior spoke eloquently to our membership last month and described how many of the patients living in the local Virginia nursing home are like family to this third-generation volunteer.

AHCA also promotes family involvement in facility-based family councils and offers advice for families in our consumer information materials. Our consumer materials can be accessed online at www.longtermcareliving.com and cover topics including:

- *Having the Conversation About Long Term Care*
- *Making the Transition*
- *Living in a Nursing Facility: the Myths and Realities*
- *Paying for Long Term Care*

Furthermore, we recognize consumer satisfaction is integral to quality facility care, which is one reason why we encourage facilities to conduct satisfaction surveys of patients, family members and staff. MIV reports that more than 4 out of 5 consumers would rate their facility as good or excellent. The survey also drills down into areas including environment, meals, staff, and solicits input as to which areas in which facilities need improvement efforts.

Transparency, Empowering Consumers & Nursing Home Compare

Long term care providers have led the healthcare sector in transparency and publicly reporting on quality. While providers continue to support transparency and public reporting of data, CMS has not successfully translated regulatory jargon, clinical descriptions, and data, into useful, accessible, and easily understandable information that consumers can use to inform their health care choices. This failing undermines the current value of *Nursing Home Compare.*

CMS' *Nursing Home Compare* website posts data collected from nursing home surveys and also lists compliance with certification requirements, progress on quality measures and indicators, and staffing data. In addition to the shortcomings as a consumer information tool, the lag time in correcting errors that are reported by providers, if a correction happens at all, is excessive. *Nursing Home Compare* also reports a facility's general staffing and patient characteristics as well as deficiencies identified in a facility's last survey. The data posted to the site does not reflect a facility's most recent survey, yet there is no explanation of that fact offered to the *Nursing Home Compare* user. While *Nursing Home Compare* has the potential to become a valuable resource, its present iteration does not empower consumers to make informed decisions about long term care options or other users of this resource.

AHCA Reform Recommendations

Mr. Chairman, the *OBRA '87* mandate was intended to move care in new directions, and it did. The law required a comprehensive assessment of each patient using a uniform Minimum Data Set (MDS) – this was groundbreaking. It was equally important that each facility needed to create and use an ongoing quality assessment and assurance committee.

This offered a platform from which each facility could evaluate the daily processes and procedures that generate positive patient outcomes. We took that direction and ran with it like no other health care sector. Even so, in the final analysis, the patient-centered, outcome-oriented, consistent system of oversight that was originally intended bears little resemblance to the reality we have today.

What we now have is a system that defines "success" and quality in a regulatory context that is often measured by the level of fines levied and the violations tallied – not by the quality of care, or quality of life, as was the original goal of *OBRA '87.*

Today, we know far more about promoting quality, and we have more tools with which to measure it than we did twenty years ago. We need to intelligently change the regulatory process to allow and encourage us to use what we have learned – to place quality over process, care over procedure, and most importantly, put patients at the forefront.

Now is the time, Mr. Chairman, to move toward such a system – a system that keeps existing oversight authority in place, and improves the universe of data used to make important decisions related to patient care. Below we identify several impediments to ongoing quality improvements and proposed solutions for consideration by this committee.

Encourage Joint Training of Surveyors & Providers

Joint training of surveyors and providers on regulations and changes to guidelines, and operational policies helps to ensure that those most directly responsible for protecting patients and providing quality care receive the same information, at the same time, and from the same source. Joint training also provides surveyors with a clearer understanding of the challenges faced daily by the staff of a nursing facility caring for these frail, elderly and disabled patients.

Greater Transparency in the QIS Pilot

The Quality Indicator Survey (QIS) pilot is currently underway in six states including, California, Connecticut, Florida, Kansas, Louisiana, and Ohio. Minnesota will be added to the pilot in early 2008, and possible use of the QIS for all facilities is still several years away. The QIS pilot is meant, in part, to provide more objective results in application of federal requirements. While we are cautiously optimistic that the QIS represents an improvement to the survey process, increased transparency regarding details of QIS from CMS is necessary for AHCA to fully support the continuation and expansion of this new system.

Eliminate the Loss of Critical Nurse Aide Training

Provisions of The Nurse Aide Training and Competency Evaluation Program prohibit a facility from offering nurse aide training as an added penalty in certain instances. Civil monetary penalties in excess of $5,000, denial of payment on new admissions, or the need for an extended or partial extended survey – which is required if surveyors find substandard quality of care (SQC) – automatically trigger a two-year suspension of a facility's nurse aide training program.

Although SQC may indicate a serious problem in a facility's care delivery system, there are times when SQC does not indicate a problem that is directly related to the care or safety of patients. The loss of a training program for two years is particularly onerous in rural areas where access to other training is extremely limited or non-existent. The loss of training is equally unfair for those receiving care in a facility. A 2004 study entitled, "Nursing Home Characteristics and Potentially Preventable Hospitalizations of Long-Stay Residents" that was published in the *Journal of the American Geriatrics Society* (Volume 52, Issue 10, pages

1730-1736), found that facilities that operate a nurses' aide training program were associated with fewer hospitalizations. Additionally, restricting training for new nurse aides, compounds the challenges long term care providers already face in recruiting and retaining high- quality caregivers—and as we are all aware, quality care is provided by those individuals at the bedside.

Furthermore, the two-year prohibition is instituted regardless of when the problem is corrected, even if the problem is corrected within a day. For example, noncompliance with the environmental aspects of regulations that have little or no impact on patient safety or quality care can trigger SQC, and therefore a two-year nurse aide training prohibition. This negatively impacts quality far more than it helps.

Remove Barriers That Threaten a Patient's Long Term Care Residence

Currently, barriers exist that prevent quality providers from stepping in and turning around a facility that is in imminent danger of closure. In these rare cases, Congress and CMS should consider the suspension of certain fines, penalties, and other enforcement actions when a facility is in "turnaround mode."

Removing such barriers would negate the need to transfer patients, who could otherwise suffer serious psychological and medical trauma from such a move, and would encourage quality providers to take over these troubled facilities.

When new leadership has stepped in to resolve a facility's chronic regulatory non-compliance, the new operator must be given a clean slate to allow time to address the root cause of the systemic noncompliance.

Alleviating the Workforce Shortage

We also urge Congress to consider the major problem of workforce in 2008 in terms of comprehensive immigration reform and developing training programs, which establish an adequate, appropriate, and well-trained domestic nurse aide workforce. We need to continue to support the *Nurse Reinvestment Act* and other federal programs that address domestic nurse supply and nursing education.

Put simply, nursing homes face major obstacles not only in terms of recruitment but also retention of nurses and certified nursing assistants (CNAs). Providing for incentives to create more nurse faculty positions will help colleges create more nursing programs, many of which are already filled to capacity. In terms of immigration, removing the caps for the recruitment of nurses from beyond our borders is an absolute necessity. We need the ability to attract sufficient nurses to the United States to fulfill our capacity. And when it comes to recruiting CNAs, we find ourselves competing with other industries altogether.

IMPROVING NURSING HOME COMPARE

We would suggest that CMS take several steps regarding *Nursing Home Compare*, including: developing specific processes for correcting erroneous data and for indicating when data is not up-to-date; conduct a focus group analysis to assess consumers' understanding of terms and data presented on *Nursing Home Compare* and how to make the site more user-friendly for consumers and other users.

TRANSPARENCY IN REPORTING – PROTECTING THE PROCESS

The long term care profession is committed to continuously improving quality of care and informing consumers about the level of care and services delivered through disclosure of quality and patient safety data. Health & Human Services (HHS) Secretary, Mike Leavitt, acknowledged that long term care has led this effort in remarks he made to the National Governors Association in August 2006. Secretary Leavitt stated,

> *"a wonderful thing is happening in the nursing home industry – they started posting their quality measures and their prices... and [because of] public disclosure of them they immediately began to improve and the price got lower and the care got better because the providers themselves said we don't want to be in a place where we are compared negatively because it will affect our market. Health care competition does work... once people have information they make good choices."*

One way to achieve quality improvement is for providers to feel confident in their ability to collect, analyze, and publish information that will lead to additional patient safety and quality assurance.

Certain patient information utilized by providers to analyze quality and safety concerns and ultimately improve clinical practice and care outcomes should be afforded more privilege and confidentiality. The information used for quality improvement purposes and the safety information should be protected from use against those providers who are committed to improving patient safety. Nursing home providers are transparent in the disclosure of quality data, but there are those who take the information and use it against us. For example, the form used by the government to document the deficiencies found during a survey—the "2567" form—is the same form where a facility records its "Plan of Correction." Submitting a Plan of Correction—required by the regulatory process—can be construed as an admission of deficient practice. Furthermore, either the state agency or CMS has given the facility a list of specifics that must be included in a Plan of Correction. The "2567" form is often used against a provide in a court case, which can seriously stymie any desire for transparency.

Voluntary and mandatory provider reporting systems that are designed to detect and disseminate patient safety and quality information should come with some hold harmless provisions as an incentive for providers willing and able to increase self-analysis and disclosure for the purposes of improving care and assuring the public of its commitment to that process.

Mr. Chairman, we ask you to help us incentivize more providers to join those who have been acknowledged by CMS and consumers for making significant advances in care and customer satisfaction. AHCA and the profession want to seize this opportunity to work with you and CMS to continue to lead the way in helping our members strive to do even more to improve care, customer satisfaction and the public trust.

CONCLUSION

Each of the areas cited above, Mr. Chairman, needs to be reformed with one goal in mind: improving patient care. We will always respect the prerogative of Congress to hold our profession accountable, yet we simply seek to implement and live by the benefits of our accumulated knowledge and proven dedication to always improving.

We pledge to work with you, Mr. Chairman, this Committee, and the entire Congress to foster an environment which continuously improves the long term care services delivered daily to nursing home patients. To this end, each of us here today seeks precisely the same objective, which is to work to improve the quality of care and quality of life for patients in America's nursing homes – and to do so in a manner that helps us best measure both progress and shortcomings.

Finally, while we are enormously proud and pleased by our quality of care and quality of life successes, we concur with all here today that there is far more to accomplish. But we must do so together.

As we can also all agree, we can best achieve the results we seek by building bridges and forging better, stronger working relationships – collaborative, open-minded relationships that look ahead to meeting the demographic challenges that await us in the near future. We owe that to every American today and in the years ahead – from every walk of life, and from every corner of our great nation. We want to accomplish this with you.

Thank you.

In: Nursing Homes Quality and Care Issues
Editor: Carlos E. Melendez
ISBN: 978-1-61668-855-4

Chapter 5

NURSING HOME TRANSPARENCY, ENFORCEMENT & QUALITY IMPROVEMENT HEARING*

Chuck Grassley

November 15, 2007

Good morning. I want to begin by thanking Chairman Kohl and the members of the Senate Special Committee on Aging for holding this important hearing. When I had the privilege of serving as chairman of this committee, many of our efforts were focused on abuse and substandard care in America's nursing homes. I'm glad to see that under the leadership of Chairman Kohl, this critical issue is remains a top priority and I applaud the committee's efforts.

In America today, there are nearly 1.7 million elderly and disabled individuals in approximately 17,000 nursing home facilities. This includes the men and women of the world war two generation – and our duty to ensure that they receive the quality care they deserve couldn't be higher.

But in addition to the Americans currently living in nursing home facilities, another issue lies on the horizon. As the baby boom generation gets older, the number of Americans in nursing home facilities is going to rise dramatically. Therefore, it's critical that we confront the issue of safe and high quality nursing home care today.

As the Ranking Member of the Senate Finance Committee, I have a special interest in nursing home care. The industry is often the subject of both my investigative and legislative work, and today I'd like to share some of my thoughts. In particular, I want to emphasize four areas that are of concern in the nursing home industry from my perspective: 1) the problem of repeat offender homes, 2) the issue of fire safety, 3) the need for greater transparency in nursing home quality, and 4) recent concern over reports that the rise of private equity firm ownership of nursing homes is resulting in poorer quality of care.

---

* This is an edited, reformatted and augmented version of a U. S. Senate Special Committee on Aging publication dated November 15, 2007.

In the nursing home industry, the vast majority of homes provide quality care on a consistent basis. They provide an invaluable service to those who can no longer care for themselves, and we applaud them for this service. But as in many sectors – this industry is given a bad name by a few bad apples that spoil the barrel. A critical tool in confronting these bad actors are the sanctions CMS can place on homes for failure to meet certain standards of care. Yet too often, nursing homes are able to "yo-yo" in and out of compliance, temporarily correcting deficiencies and having the sanctions rescinded, only to fall back into noncompliance. When sanctions *are* put in place, nursing homes currently have the incentive to file appeal after appeal, delaying the imposition of penalties and adding costs to the taxpayer. So for me the key is to ensure that nursing homes provide quality care to residents consistently – day in and day out – and if they don't, the public should be aware of that fact.

A recent GAO report examined 63 nursing homes that had been identified as having serious quality problems. Of these, nearly half continued to cycle in and out of compliance between fiscal years 2000 and 2005. 27 of the 63 homes were cited 69 times for deficiencies warranting immediate sanctions, yet in 15 of these cases sanctions were not imposed. Eight of the homes reviewed cycled in and out of compliance *seven* or more times *each* period. This is unacceptable.

But the real meaning of substandard care isn't about numbers and statistics – it's about real people – our mothers, fathers, grandparents and other loved ones. Every day there are stories reported across this nation about residents suffering or even dying from preventable situations. Imagine, just recently I read about a nursing home resident in Florida who was taken to a hospital with bed sores, a partially inserted catheter, an infected breathing tube, and maggots in one of his eyes. Each and every one of you will agree with me – *this* is unacceptable. It is an outrage.

The current system provides incentives to correct problems only temporarily and allows homes to avoid regulatory sanctions while continuing to deliver substandard care to residents. This system must be fixed. In ongoing correspondence I've had with Kerry Weems, the acting administrator of CMS, that agency has requested the statutory authority to collect civil monetary penalties sooner, to be held in escrow pending the decision on appeal. I think this is a good start. Penalties should also be meaningful – too often, they are assessed at the lowest possible amount, if at all. Penalties should be more than merely the cost of doing business; they should be collected in a reasonable timeframe; and should not be rescinded so easily. These changes will help prod the industry's bad actors to get their act together or get out of the business.

Another pressing issue is that of fire safety, and as we saw in 2003, this is an issue of life-or-death importance. That year, 16 people died in a nursing home fire in Hartford, Connecticut, and 15 died at a home in Nashville, Tennessee. Neither home had installed automatic sprinkler systems. Despite the fact that a multiple-death fire has never occurred in a sprinklered home, there are approximately 2,773 homes still without full sprinkle systems.

Following these terrible events, I requested that GAO look into the matter, and have held an ongoing conversation with CMS on how we can better protect America's nursing home residents from preventable fires. In October of 2006, CMS began to move in this direction, and expects to issue a final rule in the summer of 2008. This is a much needed improvement that will surely save lives.

While a better penalty system and better fire safety will do much to increase nursing home safety, we've also got to give nursing home residents and their families better access to information about these homes. And to do that you need more transparency.

The public currently has access to some information on nursing homes through the website "Nursing Home Compare," located on Medicare's website. Yet for all the valuable information this website provides, it could be improved through the inclusion of information on sanctions, as well as an identification of the worst offending nursing homes, often called "Special Focus Facilities." By listing these homes and the implemented enforcement actions online – information the government already has – the public would have better access to nursing home information and nursing homes would have an extra incentive to meet quality standards.

The process of choosing a nursing home is a very important and personal one for thousands of American families every year – we owe it to them to give them complete information when making this decision. Acting Administrator Weems, in a recent letter to me, gave his assurance that CMS would begin posting this information online. I thank him for his commitment and look forward to seeing this carried out. In this area, as in others, a little sunshine will go a long way.

Finally, I want to touch on an issue that has garnered a lot of attention lately – that of the purchase of nursing homes by private equity groups. Recent news reports have highlighted concerns over decreasing quality of care, decreased staffing, and decreased budgets at nursing homes purchased by private equity groups. At one home, it is alleged that 15 residents died in three years due to negligent care at a home purchased by one of these groups.

In response to these concerns, Senator Baucus and I have launched an inquiry into private equity firms and their ownership of nursing homes. Last month, we sent letters to five private equity firms asking for detailed information about their purchases and impending purchases of nursing facilities. If private equity ownership is in fact having the effect of decreased staffing, decreased budgets, and, in turn, decreased care, then something must be done about it. I plan to continue my inquiry and look forward to working with Senator Baucus to take whatever measures are appropriate in addressing this issue.

Those four issues – ineffective enforcement mechanisms, nursing home fire safety, the need for greater transparency, and concerns over private equity ownership – affect millions of vulnerable Americans and the United States Senate has a great responsibility in addressing them. Again, I thank Chairman Kohl and the members of this committee for holding this hearing, and look forward to working with you all on these matters. I also want to acknowledge the efforts of the group "Advancing Excellence in America's Nursing Homes." This group is a broad coalition of organizations dedicated to improving the quality of care and quality of life of nursing home residents. Coalitions such as this are vital to our efforts. In closing, all of us – and I mean private organizations, families, residents, caregivers, nursing home advocates, and the government – have a role to play in this important work if we want to be successful in our efforts to continue improving nursing home care. And indeed, much work remains to be done. Thank you.

In: Nursing Homes Quality and Care Issues
Editor: Carlos E. Melendez

ISBN: 978-1-61668-855-4

Chapter 6

NURSING HOME TRANSPARENCY, ENFORCEMENT & QUALITY IMPROVEMENT HEARING*

Arvid Muller

Chairman Kohl, Ranking Member Smith, and other distinguished Members of the Committee.

Thank you for giving me the opportunity to appear before you today. I am the Assisiani Direcior of Research for the Service Employees international Union (SEIU). SEIU represents almost one million health care workers, including more than 150,000 nursing home workers. SEIU respects Chairman Kohl's commitment to improving the quality of care in nursing homes. We must aiso acknowledge Senator Grassley's long-time Leadership on theses issues. And we look forward to continuing our work with both Senators on this issue. Twenty years after Congress passed landmark nursing home reform legislation, SEIU remains concerned that there are serious problems with quality of care across the industry and we fear the current enforcement systcm is simply not working. And it's difficult for families and residents to get the information they need to make an informed choice about their loved ones' care because the industry lacks transparency.

SEIU analyzes deficiency data from the Online Survey. Certification, and Reporting (OSCAR) data available from the Centers for Medicare and Medicaid Services (CMS). It's unfortunate that any way you cut the data, OSCAR shows that nursing homes have far too many quality problems. In fact, our research indicates that nursing home care overall appears to be getting even worse. In our analysis, we do not include Life safety code violations, nor did we include complaini violations. So, the total number of problems found by state inspectors in any given year was actually worse than our numbers indicate.

By compiling all the deficiencies from annual inspections for the years 2004 through 2005 we were able to determine if the number of violations per inspection increased or decreased from year to year. Unfortunately the trends we found were quite disturbing. Overail

* This is an edited, reformatted and augmented version of a U. S. Senate Special Committee on Aging publication dated November 15, 2007.

the number of violations per inspection increased each year for a total increase of 13.8% from 2004 to 2006.[i]

WHAT DO THESE DEFICIENCIES MEAN?

The next analysis we did was to look ai the severity of ine violations. Violations of resident care, (aka deficiencies) have four levels of severity.

The first, deficiencies with "potential for miriimal harm" are those that have the potential for causing no more than a minor negative impact on a resident.[ii]

Next are deficiencies with "potential for actual harm" which reflect non-compliance on the part of the nursing home in a way that causes, or has the potential to cause, no more than minimal physical, mental, or psycho-social harm to a resident.[iii]

Then there are deficiencies that "cause actual harm," causing real injury to fragile cursing home residents.[iv] Examples of actual harm citations include:

- Failure to give each resident enough fluids to keep them healthy and prevent dehydration.
- Failure to give residents proper treatment ro prevent new bed (pressure) sores or heal existing bed sores,
- Failure to make sure that residents who cannot care for themselves receive help with eating/drinking, grooming and hygiene.[v]

Finally we have deficiencies that "cause immediate jeopardy" meaning that something the nursing home did or failed to do put residents' health. safety. and lives directly in harm's way. These deficiencies require immediate comection.[vi]

Examples of immediate jeopardy citations include

- I) Failure to hire only people who have no legal history of abusing, neglecting or mistreating residents; or 2) failure to report and investigate any acts or reports of abuse: neglect or mistreatment of residents.
- Failure to protect each resident from all abuse, physical punishment. and being separated from others.[vii]

Increase from 2004	Potential for minimal harm	Potential for Actual harm	Actual harm	Immediate Jeopardy
2005	-4.3%	9.1%	8.2%	10.7%
2006	-9.6%	17.8%	19.5%	3.3%

When looked at the same data set and broke down the violations by severity we found that while the cast serious violations decreased during this time, the more serious violations increased. Violations that had only potential for minimal harm decreased from 2004 to 2006 by almost 10% However, violations that had potential for actual harm increased by 17.8% and violations that were found to have caused actual harm increased by an even greater 19.5%. Even the most serious violations, those that put the resident in immediate jeopardy increased by 3.3% per inspection.

The data for 2007 is of course still incomplete but based on about 60% of the projected inspections. the decrease in the least serious violations continues while violations that put residents in immediate jeopardy increased by over 20% from 2004.

Since the average number of violations per facilities is between six and seven during this period, we also looked at to see whether the number of facilities that had significantly more violations inereased. For this analysis we looked at all the facilities that had ten or more violations during a single inspection in any given year.[viii] We discovered an increase in the number of facilities that got cited by state inspectors for at least ten violations from 20.9% in 2004 to 26% in 2005. This means that more than one out of every four facilities inspected in 2006 had 10 or more violations of minimal federal resident care standards.

10 or more deficiencies	# of facilities surveyed	# of facilities with 10 or more	% of facilities surveyed
2004	15190	3168	20.9%
2005	14981	3603	24.1%
2006	14816	3845	26.0%

In addition, a new breed of nursing horne operator — private equity firms—has entered the nursing horne market and, for the companies we analyzed. had a clear effect on care. The private equity business model lacks trarlsparency and accountability and may be exacerbating the problems. On September 23. *The New York Times* published an investigative story on the impact on care when nursing homes are bought by private equity firms. *The New York Times* found that among other concerns with private equity ownership of nursing homes, there are serious quality of care deficiencies. In our analysis of the deficiency data, ive also looked at some of the facilities that had been hougiit by private equity firms. whose ownership structures are particularly compiex and whose business model is based on buying and selling business within a relatively short period of time. Our analysis compared the number of violations per inspection at the nursing homes for annual inspection just before they got bought by private equity to their most recent inspection. In the case of the private equity buyout of Mariner Health Care involving over 200 nursing homes and almost 30,000 beds at the end of 2504, we found that since that buy out the total number of violations increased by 29.4%: more than double the increase of the other facilities in the same states where those homes operate.

Actual harm violations increased for these same facilities increased by an incredible 66.756, while the other homes in these states saw an increase in these types of violations of 1.5%.

Deficiency Type	Mariner % Increase Post Buyout	Non-Mariner % Increase
All Deficiencies	29.4%	11.9%
Potential for Minimal Harm	-8.0%	-13.3%
Potential for Actual Harm	33.6%	18.0%
Actual harm	66.7%	1.5%
Immediate Jeopardy	87.5%	13.3%

And during their most recent inspection over 43% of this company's facilities were cited by slate inspectors for ten or more violations compared to 25% before the sale.

Facilities Cited for 10 or More Violations		
	% of Facilities Before Sale	% of Facilities After Sale
Mariner Homes	25.1%	43.8%
Non Mariner Homes	21.6%	26.2%

Most importantly, we must remember that each of these statistics reflect a fragile nursing horne resident whose needs are not met or who is or could be injured because of a nursing home's poor performance. We owe it to our seniors to do better.

The bottom line is that reform is needed to improve transparency and enforcement throughout the industry. CMS muit improve the efficiency of the enforcement system in ways that will catch the homes that need to make improvements, and they need to do so earlier in the process than many do now, before fragile nursing home residents are injured. Furthermore, given the increase in the number of homes cited for ten or more vioiations, it is imperative to focus more attention on homes that are chronic poor performers. We are encouraged that the Chairman and Senator Grassley are considering legislation to address these concerns, and we urge you to consider the following policy changes:

Increase the tranceparency and accountability of corporate ownership

- Require full disclosure to the Centers for Medicare & Medicaid Services (CMS) of all affiliated entities with a direct or indirect financial interest in the facility and their parent companies, and tile owners (including owners of the real estate), operators; and management of each facility; and require that all these entities he parties to the Medicare provider agreement and listed on Nursing Home Compare. CMS should maintain an ownership database and monitor the quality of care provided by the companies. Severe penalties. inciuding exclusion from Medicare, should be established for hiding ownership or affiliated relationships.
- CMS should address the lack of transparency by amending the provider agreement to require that providers, inciuding purchasers of an existing facility or company, deposit assets in a surety bond with the amount (to be determined) proportional to the number of beds in the facility.
- Require CMS to certify the provider agreements annually to ensure that they are consistent wilh the current ownership structure and affiliated entities.
- Require CMS to post enforcement actions against facilities and maintain actual CMS form 2565 survey reports on Nursing Home Compare.

Promote improved staffing

- Require CMS to collect electronically submitted data from facility payroll records and temporary agency contracts on a quarterly basis, including data on turnover and retention; and require CMS to report that information on Nursing Home Compare as quality measures that include a ratio of direct care nursing staff (RNs, LPNs. and CNAs) to residenis and turnover and retention rates.

- Require that information; on cost reports for Medicare be reported based on five cost centers: (1) direct care nursing services: (2) other direct care services (e.g., activities, therapies): (3) indirect care (e.g., housekeeping, dietary); (4) capital costs (e.g., building, equipment and land costs): and (5) administrative costs. The cost reports should be reported electronically to CMS and summary data should be made avaiiable on Nursing Home Compare. In 2004, MedPAC recommended requiring nursing facilities and skilled nursing facilities to publish nursing costs separately from other costs on cost reports. This recommendation was reiterated in a June 2007 MedPAC report (www.medpac.gov/Chapters/Jun07_Ch08. pdf)
- Require CMS to conduct audits of nurse staffing data reports and cost reports at least every three years to ensure the accuracy of the data reported and to prevent fraud. Severe penalties should be established for filing false reports or failing to file timely cost reports.

Taxpayers trust that Medicare and Medicaid dollars will go toward providing seniors and the disabled wirh the quality care they deserve. I thank you for inviting me here to testify about SEIU's concerns about the quality of care in nursing homes today.

End Notes

[i] The deficiency data for each year was compiled from the CMS archives of quarterl l inspection data from the Online Survey Certification and Reporting System (OSCAR). Since it sometimes takes a while for data to be submitted to CMS we combined information from multiple quarterly downloads to capture all the inspections for a particular year. We then eliminated any duplicate inspections (e.g, due to changes in provider number) and duplicate deficiencies in a single survey. Data for 2007 included deficiencies as recent as September 26th 2007 Deficiencies per inspection increased from 6.07 in 2004 to 6.90 in 2006

[ii] Centers for Medicare and Medicaid Services. State Operations Manual. "Appendix P - Survey Protocol for Long Term Care Faciiities—Part I - (Rev. 22, 12-15-06)," Section IV:D Deficiency Categorization.

[iii] Centers for Medicare and Medicaid Services. State Operations Manual. "Appendix P - Survey Protocol for Long Term Care Faciiities—Part I - (Rev. 22, 12-15-06)," Section IV:D Deficiency Categorization.

[iv] Centers for Medicare and Medicaid Services. State Operations Manual. "Appendix P - Survey Protocol for Long Term Care Faciiities—Part I - (Rev. 22, 12-15-06)," Section IV:D Deficiency Categorization.

[v] Based on information from "About the Nursing Home – Inspections," Centers for Medicare and Medicaid Services Nursing Home Compare data, downloaded 10/29/2007.

[vi] Centers for Medicare and Medicaid Services, State Operations Manual, "Appendix P - Survey Protocol for Long Term Care Facilities - Part 1 -(Rev. 22. 12-15-06)," Section 1V: Deficiency Categorization.

[vii] Based on information from "About the Nursing Home – Inspections," Centers for Medicare and Medicaid Services Nursing Home Compare data, downloaded 10/29/2007.

[viii] Even if a facility had more than one inspection that resuited in 10 violations the facility was only counted once.

In: Nursing Homes Quality and Care Issues
Editor: Carlos E. Melendez

ISBN: 978-1-61668-855-4

Chapter 7

NURSING HOME TRANSPARENCY, ENFORCEMENT & QUALITY IMPROVEMENT HEARING*

Sarah Slocum

Senator Kohl, Senator Smith and members of the Committee, thank you for the opportunity to speak with you today about nursing home transparency, enforcement and quality. Chairman Kohl, I especially want to express the appreciation of the National Association of State Ombudsman Programs for your years of work on nursing home issues and your support of the Ombudsman Program and State Survey and Certification efforts.

The landmark OBRA 1987 legislation and subsequent regulations and policies aimed at improving the quality of care and life of nursing home residents is to be celebrated. But as 20 years have passed and we still see too many instances of poor quality care and continuing poor performance by certain providers, your efforts to make improvements in this realm are much needed. Nursing homes are an awkward mix of private businesses and public funding attempting to provide care and a home-like environment for some of our most vulnerable citizens. Within this structure and given the level of vulnerability of residents, we must assure that the public has access to meaningful information about ownership, enforcement actions, financial solvency, and staffing in all certified nursing facilities.

OWNERSHIP

Congress should require the Centers for Medicare and Medicaid Services (CMS) to collect and publish information on Nursing Home Compare that shows any ownership linkages. The linkages would be determined by common ownership of the real estate, the license, or any management company operating the facility. Additionally, commonality of investors or stockholder with more than a 5% interest, and members of any board of directors or governing body should be available to Ombudsmen and consumers. CMS should also

* This is an edited, reformatted and augmented version of a U. S. Senate Special Committee on Aging publication dated November 15, 2007.

collect and publish information on ownership linkages to other businesses, such as pharmacies, laundry services, food services, etc.

Owners must be accountable to state and federal payment sources, Medicaid and Medicare, and must be required to submit audit results and financial data to demonstrate fiscal solvency of all commonly owned and related ownership entities. Further, accountability to residents should include a requirement for adequate liability insurance, so that residents who suffer wrongful death or other severe harm can pursue their private right of action in a meaningful way.

During 2005, two nursing facilities burned in Michigan. One resulted in 2 resident deaths and partial facility evacuation during the Easter holiday weekend. The other resulted in 2 resident deaths and 60 residents sent to the hospital along with complete evacuation in mid-December. There was no overt connection between these two facilities (such as the same name) and it took considerable effort by the Ombudsman to learn of their common management company. Despite different owners of the real estate, the management and operations of the two facilities were run by the same people. In both cases, inadequate staff training contributed to resident harm. Both facilities had not provided specific training and drills to assure that staff knew how and when to use fire extinguishers and fire doors. The common management company showed a pattern of inadequate training on fire safety. This is an example of how important ownership linkage information is to consumers and regulators. Had a connection been apparent, regulators could have required a review of emergency procedures in all facilities operated by this management group.

ENFORCEMENT

All enforcement actions should be published by facility name on Nursing Home Compare. Actions such as Denial of Payment for New Admissions, Civil Money Penalties, Directed Plans of Corrections, Mandatory Temporary Management, Monitors, Terminations, and Special Focus Facility status should all be clearly listed on the website. Additionally, plain English explanations of these terms must be listed after each usage of the terms so that consumers can understand the sanctions.

Residents of facilities, their loved ones, and the community at large should be notified of enforcement actions taken at facilities. Too often, Ombudsmen hear from residents and families that the termination action is their first notification of the facilities problems. Residents and families at each decertification action where I have been involved say they had no idea the facility was in such trouble. Having this information would support people in making informed decisions during nursing home placement and would give consumers and families information about areas that require vigilance in a facility. If a facility has citations about wound care, and I need that service, I may be more watchful if I have that information. Residents deserve to know.

The complete text of the survey results (the 2567 form) should also be published on Nursing Home Compare. The descriptive text of these reports helps consumers to get a better idea of what violations are cited, and what is needed to correct problems. This narrative helps consumers get a real sense of the problems in a facility, rather than just the technical regulatory description. CMS should be required to post the complete 2567, then to add information about citations overturned or modified on appeal, so that consumers have complete access to facility information.

Another essential tool for residents, families and friends is a standard complaint form. This type of form helps people who have not filed complaints before by prompting them to identify and include all basic information needed to investigate the complaint. Survey and Certification Complaint Units must also continue to provide for telephone complaints, where staff assists consumers in reducing the complaint to writing.

Additionally, local hospitals, hospice agencies, home and community based waiver programs, Area Agencies on Aging, Centers for Independent Living, the Long Term Care Ombudsman, and the Protection and Advocacy Agencies should all be directly notified of state and federal enforcement actions. These entities make referrals to nursing facilities or have clients living in these facilities. They need current and accurate information about facility status to best assist consumers.

Civil Money Penalties (CMP)

Federal CMP funds should be collected without any discount for non-appealed violations. If the violation was severe enough to merit a Civil Money Penalty, there should not be any discount. If the CMP is not correct, or is too harsh and the facility appeals the decision, the appeal process will deal with any reductions or deletions that are merited.

Federal CMP funds should be returned to the State Survey and Certification Agency where the violation took place to be used for:

- Increased staffing for survey teams and Ombudsmen;
- Funding to carry out financial viability audits and reports;
- Financial restitution to any individual resident who was harmed;
- Other quality improvement projects selected by states that provide clear and immediate benefit to residents.

Staffing

The amount and type of nursing staff (R.N.s, L.P.N.s, and C.N.A.s) serving residents in each nursing facility should be posted on Nursing Home Compare. The information should be collected by states from payroll data on a quarterly basis and audited for accuracy, then submitted to CMS. CMS should include an analysis of staffing trends by facility, and whether the facility has increased or decreased its direct care staffing levels by category over the last three years. Additionally, any substantiated complaints about staffing levels should also be listed on Nursing Home Compare.

Staffing shortages continue to plague residents and staff at many nursing facilities. A recent revisit survey at a Michigan facility resulted in a citation for Pressure Sores (F 314 based on CFR 483 .25(c)). In the narrative for this citation, an interview with a CNA, who had not turned a resident as stated in his care plan, said the following, "I have 14 residents to care for and 11 residents are total care. It's very hard to turn people every two hours because sometimes we just can't. He (Resident 56) is a two person transfer so we can't answer lights because he could fall. Nurses will turn off the light and then tell us what the resident needs which doesn't help us." Resident 56 was admitted to this facility in December 2006 with no pressure ulcers. By February 2007 he had a pressure sore on this left heel, and by September 2007 had a maggot infestation and infection that required surgery on his Stage IV pressure sore and removal of part of his heel.[1] Clearly this type of severe short staffing is unacceptable and Congress should enact safe and clearly enforceable staffing requirements to assure that no other residents suffer this fate.

Ombudsman Access to Information

All information about Ownership, Enforcement Actions, Civil Money Penalties, Staffing, and Special Focus Facilities must be shared immediately by all State Survey and Certification agencies with each State Long Term Care Ombudsman. Ombudsmen are a direct source of information for consumers, and serve as a source of counseling and information for consumers and their families and friends as they consider long term care options. Ombudsman are able to track this information, provide a sounding board for consumer questions, and help consumers understand the complex and multifaceted information they are bombarded with during what is usually a health crisis. I am deeply troubled that not all state Ombudsman have access to this information, and I urge Congress to require states and CMS to share all facility information with Ombudsmen. When Ombudsmen know about sanctions and facility status they can increase visits to safeguard resident safety and well-being. Ombudsmen also need information at the earliest possible time to be prepared to help consumers through the trauma of closure, should the facility become terminated from Medicare and Medicaid.

Ombudsmen should also be consulted in the development of the lists of potential and actual Special Focus Facilities. The data from the Ombudsman program about complaints and issues at facilities would add a consumer perspective to the decision making process around Special Focus Facilities. I urge CMS and State Survey and Certification agencies to establish and use input mechanisms to gather information from the Ombudsmen in each state.

Effect of Enforcement on Residents

For many years, the Michigan Long Term Care Ombudsman Program, and Ombudsmen in many other states, have expressed a need for CMS to hold poor performing facilities accountable, to consistently use strong enforcement action when violations exist, and to enforce all of the requirements for Quality of Care and Quality of Life found in the federal Nursing Home Reform Law of 1987. At the same time, Ombudsmen have expressed great concern over the harm suffered by residents when these same enforcement actions bring about the decertification and closure of facilities.

The Special Focus Facilities program has brought these competing concerns into sharp relief as chronically poor performing facilities receive additional scrutiny and a shortened enforcement cycle while on the Special Focus Facilities list. In Michigan, for the most part, Special Focus Facilities either improve or close. Approximately 5 facilities, slightly more than 1% of Michigan's nursing home supply, close each year in Michigan. During FY 2007, approximately 445 nursing facility residents were forced to move from their homes because of nursing home closures. The majority of these facilities were either in Special Focus status or were on the list of possible Special Focus Facilities.

Almost all of the nursing home closures in Michigan over the last 4 years have been at facilities with a high number of violations, financial problems, a higher than average percentage of their population reliant on Medicaid, and a higher than average percentage of their population made up of younger residents with largely unaddressed mental health needs. Whether the closure is labeled "Regulatory" or "Voluntary" seems largely to depend on the timing of the owner's taking action to surrender their certification, rather than on any substantive difference.

In two recent decertification actions in Michigan, the facilities have sought and received permission from CMS to voluntarily surrender their Medicare and Medicaid certification one day prior to their termination dates. The result in one case was a "Voluntary" closure. During this type of closure, the state has less control and authority over what happens to residents, the facility and corporate staff remains in charge of the building and the relocation of residents. State placement agents, ombudsmen, and community mental health agency staff are far less effective in ensuring residents' rights and choice when the facility or corporation is left in charge. These closure situations in Michigan have resulted in less resident choice about their next placement, much pressure on facility staff, residents and their families to move out quickly, and less effective state oversight during the closure. Congress should add closure provisions to federal law, so that:

- State Survey and Certification Agencies always take control of the relocation of residents during the closure;
- Special fines against owners are levied when residents are not provided meaningful choice in their next living arrangement;
- Specific timelines for each closure are established by CMS and the State Survey agency – these timelines may vary depending on the number of residents, the availability of other acceptable options and the level of risk of harm to residents remaining in the facility during the closure period;
- Federal Medicare and Medicaid payments should not be limited to thirty days after the termination date. Thirty days is often not adequate time to choose a better facility, or to transition to home and community based services. This timeline pushes residents to move to far away facilities, or to other substandard facilities in many cases.

In closing, I applaud this committee's efforts to shed light on nursing home ownership, enforcement, staffing and special focus status. Everyday I hear from consumers who are thirsty for reliable and understandable information about nursing homes. The National Association of State Ombudsman Programs stands ready to provide additional information on residents' experiences and on how information can be made accessible, transparent and meaningful to consumers. We are very grateful for your determined efforts to empower, inform and protect long term care residents.

End Notes

[1] Metron of Bloomingdale, Revisit Number Three to the Annual Survey, 11/20/2007, pp.15, 16.

In: Nursing Homes Quality and Care Issues
Editor: Carlos E. Melendez
ISBN: 978-1-61668-855-4

Chapter 8

NURSING HOME TRANSPARENCY, ENFORCEMENT & QUALITY IMPROVEMENT HEARING*

Gordon H. Smith

I want to thank Senator Kohl for holding this important hearing today to continue the discussion on nursing home quality. These discussions are necessary to ensure that those in need of longterm care get the quality care they deserve. The issue of nursing home quality and safety is of particular interest to me and I thank the panelists for being here today.

I especially want to thank Senator Grassley. As a former chair of this Committee and having served as both Chairman and Ranking Member of the Finance Committee, the interest of our citizens in nursing homes has long been a priority for him.

We know that the need for long-term care is expected to grow significantly in coming decades. Almost two-thirds of people currently receiving long-term care are over age 65, and this number is expected to double by 2030. We also know that the population over age 85, those most likely to need long-term services and supports, is expected to increase by more than 250 percent by 2040 from 4.3 million to 15.4 million.

Today, millions of Americans are receiving or are in need of long-term care services and supports. Surprisingly, more than 40 percent of persons receiving long-term care are between the ages of 18 and 64.

The past two decades have revealed a shift in the provision of long-term care. A great example of this is in my home state of Oregon, where much of the care is provided in community settings and in the recipient's home. We also have seen that long-term care providers are offering services that put the patient at the center of care, encourage inclusion of families in decision- making and give more choices in the location of the care, such as community-based and in-home settings.

As I have said in this Committee before, ensuring patient safety is a responsibility that rests with no one party or entity. It is shared by care providers, the federal and state

---

* This is an edited, reformatted and augmented version of a U. S. Senate Special Committee on Aging publication dated November 15, 2007.

governments, law enforcement agents, local agencies and community advocates. It is a responsibility that I take very seriously, as I know my colleagues do.

We must all work together more collaboratively to curb the incidence of elder abuse. We owe that to the millions of seniors who have placed their trust in our nation's long-term care system and to those who remain in their homes and in their communities. The passage of the Elder Justice Act would be a wonderful and much needed step towards this goal.

Apart from improving communication and cooperation of enforcement activities, there may need to be new, stronger policies in place to ensure that seniors receive the safest long-term care possible. I have reintroduced the "Long-Term Care Quality and Modernization Act" with Senator Lincoln. This bill encourages a number of important improvements to nursing homes and the long-term care system that aim to enhance the quality and safety of care provided to our seniors. I look forward to continuing to work with many of the advocates, industry representatives and regulators here today to ultimately pass this legislation.

I would like to applaud the work that Senator Kohl has done in this area as well, especially in regard to helping nursing homes and other facilities better identify potential bad actors in the workforce and to ensure families are informed of facility quality. It is essential that we find more effective ways to help poor performing facilities operate at a much higher level of care, or consider ways that they can be phased out of the system. We cannot let the inappropriate actions of a few continue to destroy the trust our nation's seniors have placed in the long-term care system.

I am confident that the fine panels of experts Senator Kohl has assembled today will be able to provide a fresh insight on the work that is being done at the federal, state and local levels to reduce elder abuse and provide the safest, highest quality care possible.

Thank you.

In: Nursing Homes Quality and Care Issues
Editor: Carlos E. Melendez
ISBN: 978-1-61668-855-4

Chapter 9

CMS' OVERSIGHT OF NURSING HOMES: THE SPECIAL FOCUS FACILITY & OTHER PROGRAMS TO ADDRESS TROUBLED NURSING HOMES*

Kerry Weems

Good afternoon Chairman Kohl, Senator Smith and distinguished members of the Committee. It is my pleasure to be here today to discuss the Centers for Medicare & Medicaid Services' (CMS) initiatives undertaken in the past few years to improve the quality of care for nursing home residents. Our quality efforts in this area are broad, including initiatives to enhance consumer awareness and transparency, as well as rigorous survey and enforcement processes to ensure nursing facilities provide quality care to their residents.

BACKGROUND

Americans are growing older and living longer – many with complex, chronic medical conditions. As increasing numbers of our nation's baby boom generation retire, the need for high-quality long term care, both in the community and in nursing homes will grow commensurately. About 1.5 million Americans reside in the nation's 16,400 nursing homes on any given day.[1] More than 3 million Americans rely on services provided by a nursing home at some point during the year.[2] Those individuals, and an even larger number of their family members, friends, and relatives, must be able to count on nursing homes to provide reliable care of consistently high quality.

In 2006, approximately 2.8 million (7.4 percent) of the 37.3 million persons aged 65 and over in the United States had a nursing home stay.[3] By contrast, 22 percent of the 5.3 million persons aged 85 and older had a nursing home stay in 2006. Some of these were long-term

---

* This is an edited, reformatted and augmented version of a U. S. Senate Special Committee on Aging publication dated November 15, 2007.

nursing home residents, while some had shorter stays for skilled nursing care following an acute hospitalization.[4]

Roughly 1.8 million persons received Medicare-covered care in skilled nursing facilities in 2005.[5] Medicare skilled nursing facility benefit payments increased from $17.6 billion in 2005 to nearly $21.0 billion in Fiscal Year (FY) 2007.[6] Approximately 1.7 million persons received Medicaid-covered care in nursing facilities during 2004.[7] Medical assistance payments for Medicaid-covered nursing facility services topped $47 billion in FY 2005, representing nearly 16 percent of overall medical assistance payments that year.[8]

ACTION PLAN FOR NURSING HOME QUALITY

Congress has authorized a variety of tools that enable CMS to promote – in the words of the statute – ". .the highest practicable physical, mental, and psychosocial well-being of each resident. ."[9] The most effective approach to ensure quality is one that mobilizes all available tools and aligns them in a comprehensive strategy. An internal CMS Long Term Care Task Force helps shape and guide the Agency's comprehensive strategy for nursing home quality. Each year, CMS publishes a comprehensive *Nursing Home Action Plan*[10] on our web site, which reflects the vision and priorities of the Task Force and the Agency. The current *Action Plan* outlines five inter-related and coordinated approaches – or principles of action – for nursing home quality, as described in detail below.

Consumer Awareness and Assistance

The first principle of action is consumer awareness and assistance. Aged individuals, people who have a disability, their families, friends, and neighbors are all essential participants in achieving high quality care in any health care system. The availability of relevant, timely information can significantly help such individuals to be active, informed participants in their care. This information also can increase the ability of such individuals to hold the health care system accountable for the quality of services and support that should be provided. To that end, CMS seeks to provide an increasing array of understandable information that can be readily accessed by the public.

With regard to nursing home care specifically, the CMS web site "Nursing Home Compare" at www.Medicare.gov features key information on each nursing home; the results of their three most recent quality of care inspections; and other important information for consumers, families, and friends. The web site contains the results of 19 different quality of care measures for each nursing home, such as the percent of residents who have pressure ulcers or are subject to physical restraints. Recently CMS added information to help consumers know the extent of sprinklers and other fire-safety features in each nursing home. CMS also added information about the percent of residents who were vaccinated for flu and pneumonia.

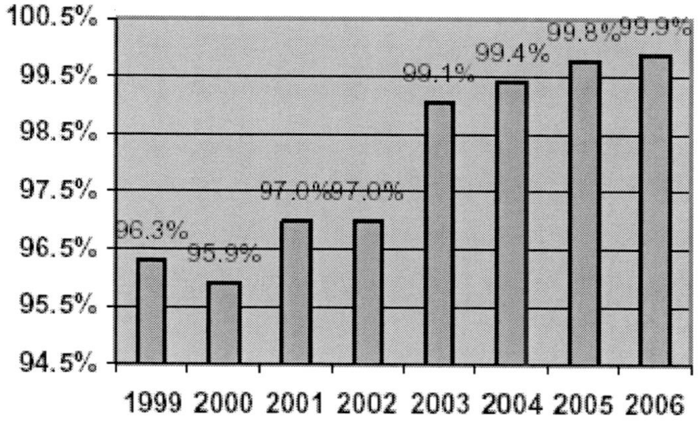

Nursing Home Surveys Percent Completed 1999-2006

Survey, Standards, and Enforcement Processes

The second principle is to have clear expectations for quality of care that are properly enforced. CMS establishes both quality of care and safety requirements for providers and suppliers that participate in the Medicare and Medicaid programs. Such requirements are carefully crafted to highlight key areas of quality and convey basic, enforceable expectations that nursing homes must meet. More than 4,000 Federal and State surveyors conduct on-site reviews of every nursing home at least once every 15 months (and about once a year on average). CMS also contracts with quality improvement organizations (QIOs) to assist nursing homes to make vital improvements in an increasingly large number of priority areas.

We take our responsibilities for on-site surveys of nursing homes seriously. In 2006, the most recent year for which complete data are available, the percent of nursing homes that were surveyed at least every fifteen months reached 99.9 percent – the highest rate ever recorded. In addition to about 16,000 comprehensive surveys that year, CMS and States conducted more than 45,000 complaint investigations in nursing homes. Our strengthened fire-safety inspections led to the identification of 67.8 percent more deficiencies in 2006 compared to 2002 (to 66,470 from 39,618). Nursing homes are responding to these findings by improving their fire-safety capability as never before.

Quality Improvement

The third *Nursing Home Action Plan* principle is to have effective quality improvement strategies. CMS is promoting a program of quality improvement in a number of key areas. These areas include reduction in the extent to which restraints are used in nursing homes; reduction in the prevalence of preventable pressure sores that threaten the health and well-being of a significant number of nursing home residents; and the Agency's participation in a larger national movement known as "culture change." Culture change principles echo Omnibus Budget Reconciliation Act (OBRA) of 1987 principles of knowing and respecting each nursing home resident in order to provide individualized care that best enhances each person's quality of life. The concept of culture change encourages facilities to change outdated practices to allow residents more input into their own care and encourages staff to serve as a team that responds to what each person wants and needs.

Quality through Partnerships

The fourth *Nursing Home Action Plan* principle is to promote quality through enthusiastic partnerships with any and all organizations that will join with us. No single approach or actor can fully assure quality. CMS must mobilize and coordinate many actors and many techniques through a partnership approach. State survey agencies and the QIOs under contract with CMS are more than ever coordinating their distinct roles so as to achieve better results than could be achieved by any one actor alone. CMS is also a founding member of the "Advancing Excellence in America's Nursing Homes" campaign. This campaign is an exceptional collaboration among government agencies, advocacy organizations, nursing home associations, foundations, and many others to improve the quality of nursing homes across the country.[11] The campaign voluntarily enlists nursing homes to measure and make improvements in eight key quality of care areas. More than 6,000 nursing homes have signed up to make quality improvements such as the consistent assignment of staff to individual nursing home residents; the assessment of satisfaction on the part of residents and families; or the reduction of pressure ulcers.

Value-Based Purchasing

The fifth principle of the *Nursing Home Action Plan* is to use purchasing power to promote quality. As the largest third-party purchasers of nursing home services in the country, States and CMS exert leverage to insist on basic levels of quality. CMS is working collaboratively with private and public organizations to stimulate high quality care and improve efficiency. Payment reforms could show promise in helping providers deliver care that prevents complications, avoids unnecessary medical services, and achieves better outcomes at a lower overall cost.

With these five principles in mind, the testimony will now turn to two topics that we understand may be of special interest to the Committee. The first is the issue of nursing home ownership, and the second is the CMS "Special Focus Facility" initiative.

Nursing Home Ownership

CMS is aware of recent media reports about the relationship between quality nursing home care and nursing home ownership, particularly investor-owned facilities. We understand the importance of responsible ownership of nursing facilities serving the Medicare and Medicaid population. To that end, in response to these recent concerns CMS is actively engaged in improving the transparency of facility ownership by working collaboratively with nursing home providers.

CMS has developed a new system called the Provider Enrollment Chain and Ownership System (PECOS). This new system is designed to track and maintain improved information regarding entities that own five percent or more of a nursing home and to ensure only eligible providers and suppliers are enrolled and maintain enrollment in the Medicare program. The primary function of the provider enrollment application is to gather information from a provider or supplier that tells CMS who it is; whether it meets State licensing qualifications and federal quality of care and safety requirements to participate in Medicare; where it practices or renders its services; the identity of the owner of the enrolling entity; and information necessary to establish the correct claim payment. The PECOS database is being populated now and is expected to be 70 percent populated by the second quarter of FY 2008. Supported by this new system, CMS will be able to better track ownership, potentially beginning in the Spring of 2008. CMS also is exploring a web-based application for 2008 to allow providers and suppliers to enter contact information and other updates directly. This will facilitate the ability of nursing homes to maintain up-to-date enrollment information.

In terms of quality, CMS focuses on the quality of care experienced by residents regardless of who owns the facility. Our focus on actual outcomes ensures that Medicare's quality assurance system does not depend on any theory of quality or theory of ownership. Instead, the federal survey and certification system is grounded in what CMS and State nursing home surveyors actually find through on-site inspection; through in-person interviews with residents and staff; through the eyewitness observation of care processes; and through the review of records of care. CMS continuously seeks to improve the effectiveness of both the survey process and the enforcement of quality of care requirements. An example of such continuous improvement is our Special Focus Facility initiative that addresses the issue of nursing homes that persist in providing poor quality.

Special Focus Facility Program

The Special Focus Facility program was initiated because a number of facilities consistently provided poor quality care, yet periodically fixed a sufficient number of the presenting problems to enable them to pass one survey, only to fail the next survey. Moreover, they often failed the next survey for many of the same problems as before. Such facilities with an "in and out" or "yo-yo" compliance history rarely addressed the underlying systemic problems that were giving rise to repeated cycles of serious deficiencies.

Nursing homes on the Special Focus list represent those with the worst survey findings in the country, based on the most recent three years of survey history. The selection methodology takes into account for the severity of deficiencies and the number of deficiencies. Deficiencies identified during complaint investigations are also included in the computation. Each State selects its Special Focus nursing homes from a CMS candidate list of approximately 15 eligible nursing homes in their own State, using additional information available to the State regarding the nursing homes' quality of care in order to make the final selection.

States conduct twice the number of standard surveys for Special Focus nursing homes compared to other nursing homes. If serious problems continue then CMS applies progressive enforcement until the nursing home either (a) graduates from the Special Focus program because it makes significant improvements that last; or (b) is terminated from participation in the Medicare and Medicaid programs; or (c) is given more time due to a trendline of improvement and promising developments, such as sale of the nursing home to a new owner with a better track record of providing quality care.

To analyze the impact of the Special Focus Facility initiative CMS compared the 128 nursing homes selected in 2005 with alternate nursing homes on the candidate list that were not selected. The Special Focus nursing homes had more deficiencies than others: 11 deficiencies on average in the Special Focus Facilities compared with 9 deficiencies for the alternates and 7 for nursing homes on average. However, over the course of the next two years approximately 42 percent of the Special Focus nursing homes had significantly improved to the point of meeting the Special Focus Facility graduation criteria, whereas only 29 percent of the alternates had so improved. At the same time, change of ownership or closure of poorly performing nursing homes was greater in the Special Focus nursing homes. Approximately 15 percent of the Special Focus nursing homes were terminated from participation in Medicare compared with less than 8 percent in the alternates and 2 percent for all other nursing homes. The better response of the Special Focus nursing homes in addressing deficiencies has been a function of the greater attention that CMS paid to those nursing homes on the Special Focus Facility list, and the imperative for action that is built into the Special Focus Facility program design.

The Special Focus initiative can pay great quality-of-care dividends for nursing home residents. For example, a nursing home in rural Monck's Corner, South Carolina, was a Special Focus nursing home that failed to improve significantly over the 18 months after it was first selected. As a result, in April 2007 CMS issued a Medicare notice of termination to the facility. We were prepared to see the 132 nursing home residents relocated to other facilities that provided better care. At that point, however, the nursing home operators evidenced a willingness to implement the type of serious reforms that had clear potential to transform their quality of care. CMS agreed to extend the termination date provided the nursing home would enter into a legally-binding agreement to institute certain quality-focused reforms. We required that they undergo a root cause analysis of their underlying systems-of-care deficiencies, to be conducted by a QIO selected by CMS. We required that the nursing home then develop an action plan based on the root cause analysis, and also place $850,000 in escrow to pay for the reforms indicated by the action plan and root cause analysis. These interventions were successful. The nursing home passed the subsequent survey, was purchased by another owner, and is on track to graduate from the Special Focus Facility initiative provided it can sustain the improvements over time. The corporation that operated the nursing home is now seeking to replicate this approach with other nursing homes that it operates

CONCLUSION

Mr. Chairman, thank you for the opportunity to testify here today. Regardless of setting or ownership, quality health and long-term care for Medicare and Medicaid beneficiaries is of the utmost importance to CMS. To that end, I plan to work to ensure high quality medical care for all nursing home residents. I would be pleased to address any questions or hear any comments you may have.

End Notes

[1] Centers for Medicare & Medicaid Services. *2007 Action Plan for (Further Improvement of) Nursing Home Quality* (www.cms.hhs.gov/SurveyCertificationGenInfo/downloads/2007ActionPlan.pdf) at i.
[2] *Ibid.*
[3] Centers for Medicare & Medicaid Services. *Nursing Home Data Compendium* (http://www.cms.hhs.gov/CertificationandComplianc/12 _NHs.asp#TopOfPage).
[4] *Ibid.*
[5] U.S. Department of Health and Human Services. *2007 CMS Statistics* at 4 and 34. Washington D.C.: U.S. Government Printing Office.
[6] *2007 CMS Statistics* at 3 and 28.
[7] *2007 CMS Statistics* at 4 and 39. "Nursing facility" in this context includes SNFs and all other nursing facilities other than intermediate care facilities (ICF/MR).
[8] *2007 CMS Statistics* at 29. Note these figures exclude payments under SCHIP.
[9] Section 1819(b)(2) of the Social Security Act.
[10] See http://www.cms.hhs.gov/CertificationandComplianc/12 NHs.asp#TopOfPage
[11] Information about the campaign for *Advancing Excellence in America's Nursing Homes* may be found at: http://www.nhqualitycampaign.org

In: Nursing Homes Quality and Care Issues
Editor: Carlos E. Melendez
ISBN: 978-1-61668-855-4

Chapter 10

NURSING HOME TRANSPARENCY, ENFORCEMENT & QUALITY IMPROVEMENT HEARING*

Bonnie Zabel

INTRODUCTION

Chairman Kohl, Ranking Member Smith and members of the Committee, I am pleased to have the opportunity to testify today on behalf of Marquardt Memorial Manor (Marquardt Manor) and the American Association of Homes and Services for the Aging (AAHSA), of which we are a member. Marquardt Manor is also a member of the Wisconsin Association of Homes and Services for the Aging (WAHSA), where I serve on the Board of Directors.

The members of the American Association of Homes and Services for the Aging (www.aahsa.org) serve as many as two million people every day through mission-driven, not-for-profit organizations dedicated to providing the services people need, when they need them, in the place they call home. Our 5,700 members offer the continuum of aging services: adult day services, home health, community services, senior housing, assisted living residences, continuing care retirement communities and nursing homes. AAHSA's commitment is to create the future of aging services through quality people can trust.

Marquardt Manor is a certified Medicare and Medicaid skilled nursing facility. Founded in 1969, Marquardt Manor is a part of Marquardt Village, a retirement community sponsored by the Western District of the Moravian Church. Our mission is to care for the elderly and the handicapped in a Christian environment, although we are open to all faiths. The Marquardt retirement complex began as the nursing home but now consists of all levels of services and housing – low-income and market rate senior housing; assisted living; skilled nursing; supportive home care services; home health; therapy; hospice; and a senior center.

I joined Marquardt Manor 20 years ago as a nurse and was appointed administrator in 1994. Our residents receive a wide range of medical and social services, but we are more than

* This is an edited, reformatted and augmented version of a U. S. Senate Special Committee on Aging publication dated November 15, 2007.

medical services, we are home for our residents. Quality of care and quality of life merge in three specific ways:

- We care about our resident's transition to Marquardt and quality of care. We are fully prepared before we accept a resident – we tell hospital discharge planners that we require a full and complete medical history so that we are prepared with the correct medication, correct immediate care plan, and correct immediate treatment when a new resident arrives. Care happens immediately – a personalized care plan needs to be in place upon admission.
- We care about our residents' comfort. Although we are almost 70% Medicaid funded, each of our rooms is private and carpeted, with its own bath. Residents are encouraged and able to bring their personal furnishings so that they can say, especially if they will be with us for a long time, "I am home". While the overhead for private rooms is higher than shared rooms, the benefits far outweigh the costs: residents are more content and relate better to each other; families and kids visit more often and have much better visits. On the care side, infections have been reduced; nurses have more time to spend with each resident; rooms stay much cleaner; and everyone is much happier. Creating a good atmosphere is not a frivolous activity, it is central to a good and caring environment.
- We care about our workforce. We have almost no turnover and we are an employer of choice in our community. Our staffing levels are higher than average (3.9 hours per resident) as is our pay (starting salary for CNAs is $13.95 per hour plus benefits, compared with $9.00 in Milwaukee and Madison), and we have excellent in-house education and training programs. We created an educational program with our local high school which has funneled interested and well-trained young people into our field as CNAs. They get their on-the-job training at Marquardt Manor as they are completing their high school education. Our turnover really is related to graduates who decide to move on, often to get advanced degrees – we are proud that we have educated generations of young people to join our field and provide quality care throughout Wisconsin and the country.

  In addition we have and enforce fair and reasonable work rules – good work is recognized and poor quality not tolerated. We recognize the value of our workforce through a program we developed called "Gratitude, Attitude", which is now being promoted statewide by WAHSA, where staff and residents share appreciations for each other. Staff feel that their work is recognized, and residents can express what really matters to them in their every day life (taking a walk, having their hand held, morning bath – the "little" things that aren't medical but are essential and personal) which in turn helps us provide better service.

  Finally, we care about our employees as people – we recognize that balancing work and family is not easy and have created informal and formal programs to help our staff. We provide in-service programs for staff in such areas as coping skills and balancing work and family. Personally, I have an open door – staff knows that they can come to me with concerns and that we will work together for solutions.

In my testimony today, I will focus on our field's efforts to improve nursing home transparency and quality, and address certain improvements to the overall system that could improve the consumer's ability to make informed decisions regarding the decision to enter a nursing home.

TRANSPARENCY

It is difficult for consumers to obtain adequate and useful information on nursing homes so that they can make an informed decision for themselves or a loved one. The information that is available is not written for the lay person and does not contain critical information to assess the quality of life and care provided by the home. This lack of good information is particularly disturbing because consumers seldom have the time or capacity to research homes.

The primary source of information is Nursing Home Compare, the website established and maintained by CMS. Nursing Home Compare contains the results of the latest surveys for each Medicare and Medicaid-certified nursing home, quality measures based on the information collected for the Minimum Data Set (MDS) Repository, and some general information regarding each nursing home. Although an effort has been made to explain each reported measure and deficiency citation, the site never actually explains the process and the meaning of the results, how surveys are conducted, what they mean and don't mean. How should the consumer assess the meaning of a deficiency that ranks as a "2" and affects a "few" residents? Consumers cannot even determine if cited deficiencies relate to many incidents or one incident. Nor is there any lay explanation of the facts underlying the deficiency so that a consumer can understand the meaning of the deficiency. What is the actual impact on "quality"? How should the consumer use this data? Other issues that have been raised about the information provided on Nursing Home Compare relate to the reliability of the data[1], as well as understanding that compliance with regulations is not the same thing as quality.

None of these questions is answered, even though understanding how to interpret survey data and integrate this data into one's analysis of any particular nursing home seems like fairly basic information.

In Wisconsin, the state has developed its own website, (http://dhfs.wisconsin.gov /bqaconsumer/NursingHomes/CIRindex.htm), using the same data, but presented in a more consumer-friendly manner. The reports are re-titled "Consumer Information Reports" (CIR) and contain explanations of the information reported in plain English. In addition, the CIR contains useful information on staffing retention and turnover rates. Staffing is one of the key indicators for quality. A home with a low turnover and high retention of staff is more likely to have higher quality and greater satisfaction of staff and residents, and so this information can be very useful to consumers.

The survey is only one tool for evaluating a nursing home, indeed it may be the least useful in the end because it only reports on deficiencies and does not provide information on all the other elements of care and services that are critical for evaluating quality of care. Unfortunately, there really is no other data source for identifying which nursing homes have high quality.[2] As a result, everyone from CMS to consumer groups to nursing homes ourselves urge prospective residents or their decision makers to visit the nursing homes they are considering if at all possible. . The time to visit prospective homes and the tools to analyze the information obtained from NH Compare and their visits, are critical to the ability of consumers to make thoughtful and intelligent decisions.

There are several variations of tools for consumers. CMS has developed a "Guide to Choosing a Nursing Home" (which unfortunately is buried deep in its website but which can be found on the home page of the Wisconsin site). AAHSA has also developed a publication for consumers, "How to Choose a Nursing Home", http://www.aahsa.org/consumer_info/how_to_choose/tour_nursing_home.asp.[3] Each of these guides tries to provide the consumer with questions that will hopefully elicit sufficient information to identify the quality of the care and services provided.

In addition, AAHSA developed and recommends that our members distribute two checklists to prospective residents and their families, The Consumers Guide to Quality Aging Services (http://www.aahsa.org/qualityfirst/asse ssment/documents/consumers _guide.pdf) and a checklist called "First Impressions" which is designed to provide feedback to the provider but also serves as a good one-page checklist for consumers themselves. (http://www.aahsa.org/qualityfirst/resources/public_trust/documents/FirstImpression.pdf)

The Consumers Guide to Quality Aging Services is considerably different than the standard guides because it tracks the elements of AAHSA's Quality First initiative.[4] The AAHSA Guide recommends that the prospective consumer ask the nursing home questions such as: "Does your organization participate in a quality improvement or accreditation program (and if so, explain which one and why)"; "Who serves on your Board of Directors?"; "How does your organization identify and adopt new care and services practices?"; "What kinds of community programs or services do you bring into the facility, and how do you involved residents in programs, activities and events in the neighboring community?"; "Is your staff encouraged to give feedback? For example, do you conduct staff satisfaction surveys and if so, how do you use the results?", and "What is the average length of employment for your staff members and what reasons do employees cite for leaving your organization?"

AAHSA linked several questions in the Consumers Guide to "Governance and Accountability", one of the elements of AAHSA Quality First, because good governance and corporate accountability are critical to quality. Not-for-profits are not only obligated to report to the public on their finances, they are also legally and morally obligated to reinvest their earnings in their community, whether by providing more and better services, higher pay for staff, improving the physical environment or serving more people, to name just a few possibilities.[5]

Consumers and Choice: The Challenge of Transition

One of the most pressing problems for consumers is having the time to use the various tools available. Nursing home admissions through Medicare by definition have to be preceded by a 3- day hospital stay and it is has been our experience that most nursing home admissions in fact come directly from hospitals. Thus, the gatekeeper tends to be the hospital discharge planner. A number of commentators have examined the transition process from hospital to nursing home and identified a considerable number of concerns, including failure to provide x-rays and other studies, failure to include end of life documents (do not resuscitate orders), dietary information and the like when patients are transferred to nursing homes.[6]

The ability of the consumer/caregiver/patient to make careful choices is likewise compromised. As hospital stays have shortened, the time between admission and discharge planning has likewise shortened, thus reducing the ability of the caregiver to make careful choices. The National Alliance for Caregiving has published a pamphlet for caregivers explaining the process and providing advice on how to manage and challenge decisions,[7] but it is unlikely that many consumers have access to this document. Family and patient may feel they have no choice but to take the recommendation/order of the hospital – and no meaningful time to determine alternatives much less search for information on quality of care and life and then seek out the best facilities.

These transitions, we firmly believe, need to be addressed if we are serious about wanting consumers to exercise choice based on meaningful information and if we want the people we care for to move through the system smoothly. AAHSA has joined with 26 other organizations to form The National Transitions of Care Coalition (NTOCC), which brings together thought leaders, health care providers and consumers from various care settings to address improving the quality of care coordination and communication when individuals are transferred from one level of care to another.

Quality Initiatives from the Field

AAHSA and many of our members have developed and implemented initiatives to improve both the quality of care and the quality of life of people living in nursing homes. AAHSA's own "five big ideas for the future of aging services" include cultural transformation: the creation of a healthy nursing home workplace based on respect for caregivers, team building and management, continuous quality improvement, and resident centered care.

A few examples of quality initiatives in which our members have taken a leading role[8]:

Pioneer Network

Ten years ago, nursing home leaders who wanted to change the dynamics of our field to reflect life and growth began meeting together to find common areas for research and reform. The Pioneer Network was established in 2000 as the umbrella organization for the culture change movement. Its members work with long-term care professional organizations, facilities and their staffs in implementing fundamental changes in the operations of nursing facilities. Several AAHSA conferences have included educational sessions led by Pioneer Network members. Nursing homes that have implemented Pioneer principles are reporting improved staff retention and resident outcomes. Nine states have formed culture change coalitions. The Network has now expanded to include providers of home- and community-based services.

Wellspring

Wellspring, an initiative begun by a group of AAHSA members in Wisconsin in 1994, integrates federal quality indicators, best practices and a new management paradigm to dramatically improve resident outcomes and cost efficiency. Fundamental to the Wellspring program is the concept that the definition of quality care is created by top management, but that the best decisions about how the care is delivered to each resident are made by the front-line staff who knows the residents best. This empowerment is achieved through extensive line staff education in the form of "care resource teams", shared decision-making and enhancing critical thinking skills of all staff. The program is lead by a geriatric nurse consultant who utilizes other clinical experts for teaching best practices.

Group process is central to Wellspring. The shift from traditional autocratic management structure to staff empowerment where frontline staff has equal responsibility for resident outcomes is what has made Wellspring unique. Key components are establishing permanent staff assignments to groups of residents and allowing staff to do their own scheduling.

Because of the initial success Wellspring achieved (98% resident/family satisfaction, a cut in the CNA turnover rate from 105% to less than 30%, a waiting list of CNA applicants, high staff retention, and good survey results) the program now is being replicated in nursing homes in several states.

Eden Alternative

Several years ago, Dr. Bill Thomas began a program to combat the loneliness, helplessness and boredom that many nursing home residents experienced. His program has now been replicated across the country, and participating nursing homes commit to creating human habitats, with residents at the center, surrounded by plants, animals and children. Elders in these communities have the opportunity to both give and receive care, to engage in meaningful activity, and to experience variety and spontaneity.

A vital part of the Eden Alternative is the de-emphasis on top-down bureaucratic authority, seeking instead to place the maximum possible decision-making authority into the hands of the elders or into the hands of those closest to them.

Green Houses

Green Houses, also the brainchild of Dr. Thomas, build on the concepts of the Eden Alternative. These projects emphasize small communities for elders and staff where necessary medical care is provided, but is not the focus of activity. The Green House is intended to replace large institutions with small, social settings for six to ten elders. Elders have private rooms and baths, situated around a common kitchen and dining area. Elders have access to outdoor gardens and patios and can choose their own activities throughout the day without the imposition of any kind of sleeping or eating schedule. Green House projects now are being planned or operated in eighteen states.

Advancing Excellence in America's Nursing Homes

Advancing Excellence in America's Nursing Homes is a two year, coalition-based campaign concerned with how we care for elderly and disabled citizens. This voluntary campaign:

- Monitors key indicators of nursing home care quality
- Promotes excellence in caregiving for nursing home residents
- Acknowledges the critical role nursing home staff have in providing care

The campaign builds on the success of other quality initiatives like Quality First, the Nursing Home Quality Initiative (NHQI), and the culture change movement. Campaign goals include creating a culture of person-centered, individualized care and an empowered workforce in nursing homes. The campaign has brought together all long-term care stakeholders, including consumer advocates, medical and quality improvement experts, and enforcement agency officials.

Several thousand nursing homes already have enrolled and committed to working on three out of eight quality indicators: reducing high risk pressure ulcers, reducing the use of daily physical restraints, improving pain management for short-stay, post-acute patients and for longer term nursing home residents, establishing individual targets for improving quality, assessing resident and family satisfaction with the quality of care, increasing staff retention; and improving consistent assignment of nursing home staff, so that residents regularly receive care from the same caregivers.

Quality First

The Quality First initiative, begun in 2002, is a philosophy of quality and a framework for earning public trust in aging services. More important, it is a renewal of our commitment as aging- services providers to help older adults and their loved ones live their lives to their fullest potential. Through Quality First, we work in partnership with all stakeholders - government, consumers and the people we serve and their families - to create quality of care and quality of life in aging services.

AAHSA Quality First provides all AAHSA members with opportunities to reaffirm their public commitment to quality; assess their strengths and opportunities for improvement; pursue continuous quality improvement based on the belief that improvement is always possible; and earn the public's trust and the confidence of consumers. A majority of our members have signed the Quality First covenant, and we encourage all of our members to use the tools provided for assessment of areas in which services may be improved.

Center for Aging Services Technology (CAST)

The application of technology to aging services is one of AAHSA's "five big ideas" for the future of aging services. A few years ago, we established the Center for Aging Services

Technologies, which has brought together researchers, technology companies, and long-term care providers to develop and apply technological solutions to aging services issues. These initiatives promise greater efficiency and quality in service delivery at the same time that they will give consumers more choices in the services they may obtain and the settings in which they receive them.

Responses to the Challenges Related to the Workforce Crisis

Adequate staffing is a challenge that will not go away for the foreseeable future. The nursing home reform provisions of OBRA '87 contain no set levels of staffing, and the statute's general prescription that staffing must be sufficient for residents to attain and maintain their highest practicable level of functioning has been criticized as inadequate. However, the most recent staffing study by the Centers for Medicare and Medicaid Services concluded that there was insufficient data on which to base and recommend specific staffing levels for nursing facilities. In addition, nursing homes face the same nursing shortage that prevails throughout the healthcare field, and are at a competitive disadvantage as compared to other health care providers in recruiting and retaining the staff they and their residents need.

A recent report to the National Commission for Quality Long-Term Care by the Institute for the Future of Aging Services describes the workforce crisis in the long-term care field and makes a number of recommendations for meeting this challenge. The report lists the need to bring more people into the long-term care field, to provide more competitive wages and benefits, to improve working conditions and job quality, to make larger and smarter investments in education and workforce development, to develop new models of service delivery and to moderate the demand for hands-on care through the application of technology.

AAHSA is working on all of these fronts. We encourage our nursing home members to open their doors to nursing schools and to offer opportunities for rotation through their facilities. We have also supported the concept of career ladders for nursing assistants to enter the field of professional nursing. Since 1989, under a grant from the Patient Care Division of Proctor and Gamble, we have sponsored an annual scholarship program for nursing assistants to become RNs or LPNs. In addition, we have many nursing facility members who have independently developed scholarship or tuition assistance programs to enable nurse aides under their employ to become registered (RNs) or licensed practical nurses (LPNs). Marquardt Manor partnered with the local high school in Watertown to train students to become CNAs, using our home for on the job training.

To address the issue of job quality, the Institute for the Future of Aging Services has undertaken the national Better Jobs Better Care campaign and several other initiatives to research and demonstrate organizational changes that make nursing homes attractive places to work.

Congress also has a role to play in growing staffing resources in our field. The Nursing Workforce Development programs under Title VIII of the Public Health Service Act educate nurses, enable them to remain current with developments in their field and enhance their ability to supervise other staff. The programs also include loans to increase the number of qualified faculty at nursing schools, which have had to turn away thousands of applicants for nursing education due to faculty shortages. These programs have been flat-funded for the last several years as the nursing shortage continues to grow. Additional resources are essential to meet the rising need for nursing care, and we urge an increase in funding to $200 million for these programs in fiscal 2008.

Furthermore, the IFAS report noted the need for more parity in wages and benefits between acute and long-term care settings. Because approximately seventy percent of the cost of nursing home care is paid under Medicare and Medicaid, governmental payment policies disproportionately influence the amount of resources that nursing homes have available to compensate their staff. The Long-Term Care Quality Improvement Act, H.R. 1166, introduced in the House during the last Congress, would have required the Department of Health and Human Services to study the adequacy of the entire package of funding for long-term care, Medicaid as well as Medicare.

This legislation, reintroduced in the 110th Congress as H.R. 3784, calls for nursing homes to report separately on their Medicare cost reports the amounts they spend on wages and benefits for nursing staff, by staff level, breaking out the figures for registered nurses, licensed professional nurses, and certified nurse assistants. Since staffing is so integral to quality of care, AAHSA felt that this requirement would be a strong first step toward aligning payment incentives with quality. Under current policies, Medicare pays for skilled nursing at the same rate whatever the quality of care provided. We understand that CMS is beginning to develop policies to tie payment incentives to quality and we welcome this initiative.

In addition, the IFAS report noted that the negative public perception that is fostered through the media and sensational reports that focus only on the harmful incidents and occurrences in nursing facilities is demoralizing to front-line workers. We recognize and concur that incidents of bad care are intolerable. However, the kind and compassionate care that is provided on a daily basis by the vast majority of nursing home staff members goes without notice. Portraying the entire nursing home profession in a negative light is unfair to the many dedicated staff who work continuously to assure quality care to the residents they serve. Not only does this do a disservice to these individuals, but it results in a chilling effect on our ability to recruit and retain competent, caring individuals. The long-range impact of "negative-only publicity" on our organizations is inestimable.

Recommendations

We believe the nursing home reform provisions of OBRA '87 have led to significant improvements in the quality of nursing home care. However, as implemented the federal survey and certification system fails to give consumers a reliable means of choosing the best nursing home care for themselves or their loved ones. Inconsistency in survey results and the imposition of remedies with a limited right of appeal may cause consumers to avoid facilities that in fact are providing good care. In addition, CMS's efforts to improve state inspections and enforcement and crack down on poor performers still fail to target bad providers, as noted in a recent GAO report (GAO-07-241). Oversight authorities must expend the same amount of time and resources on facilities with exemplary records as they do on those demonstrating chronic or serious quality of care problems, and facilities that consistently fail to provide appropriate quality of care remain in business.

Specifically, we recommend

Nursing Home Compare should be revamped to ensure that the information provided is accurate, reliable and understandable to consumers. The site should contain clear explanations of the survey process, what deficiencies mean in plain English and an explanation of the rating system. Information that shows the provider corrected the deficiency would be helpful. In addition, the site should explain the difference between compliance, i.e., that the facility has met the minimum standards at the time of the inspection, and quality. Finally, the "Guide to Choosing a Nursing Home" should be clearly linked on the home page. CMS could consider linking to other organizations' publications as the Wisconsin website does.

The importance of transitions – in particular from hospital to nursing home – needs to be addressed in a constructive fashion. Ensuring that patients and their families have sufficient information and time to make a decision is critical, as well as ensuring that nursing facilities receive all the information they need from the hospital in a timely fashion.

Part of transparency and accountability is to understand where Medicare dollars are going. H.R. 3784 mandates reporting of expenditure broken out by type of staff, and AAHSA urges support for this measure.

We believe that while OBRA '87 has led to significant improvements in the quality of nursing home care, some provisions of the statute no longer meet the needs of today's nursing home consumer.

The nursing assistant shortage has compounded the counter-productivity of OBRA's two-year disqualification of nurse-aide training programs for facilities found to be out of compliance with certain standards. An inability to train nurse aides, once compliance has been achieved and demonstrated, results in a potential compromise to quality of care that is inappropriate and unnecessary, and is addressed in S. 1980, introduced by Sen. Smith.

Barriers to the takeover of poor performers by new owners with good records of compliance should be removed. Under the current system, a facility's compliance record and any enforcement remedies sustained by a previous owner are required to be transferred to the new owner. This forces competition between the new owner's resources to restore quality of care and services to the residents, and the previous owners' liabilities related to compliance and financial penalties. Faced with carryover liability for heavy fines by a consistently poor performer, healthier facilities are unlikely to step in to try to turn a problem facility around. In areas where long-term care services are limited, residents may have few or no alternatives to remaining in a poor facility, and facilitating new management would be in the residents' best interests.

The existing mandate that states use civil monetary penalty funds to improve resident care must be better enforced; many states have not adopted programs to implement this requirement and the monies collected are being used for other purposes. To fulfill the mandate, CMP funds should be used for surveyor training, consultation and technical assistance to facilities in developing and implementing quality improvement or resident care protocols.

America's seniors and their families need a quality assurance system that enables them to choose facilities that provide excellent quality of care and quality of life. An approach must be developed that allows surveyors and care-giving staff to work not only on promoting and achieving sustained compliance, but on meeting individual care needs and expectations to improve care. Nursing home care is evolving, and we need a resident-focused system that fosters continuous quality improvement. The focus of the survey and enforcement process should be on fixing problems and offering expert guidance rather than on punishment.[9]

CONCLUSION

It is appropriate for all stakeholders to take stock of the progress that has been achieved in improving care and services provided by our nursing homes and the ways in which the highest quality nursing home care can be ensured and achieved for the oldest and most vulnerable Americans. It is incumbent upon all of us – government, providers, community – to make sure that consumers have reliable information to select the best nursing homes, and the time and ability to use that information.

AAHSA commits itself and its members to continuous improvement in the quality of care and services we provide, and we look forward to working with the Senate Special Committee on Aging to ensure continued progress in our field.

RELIABILITY OF THE NURSING HOME SURVEY PROCESS: A SIMULTANEOUS SURVEY APPROACH

Robert H. Lee, PhD,[1] Byron J. Gajewski, PhD,[3] and Sarah Thompson, PhD[2]

Purpose: We designed this study to examine the reliability of the nursing home survey process in the state of Kansas using regular and simultaneous survey teams. In particular, the study examined how two survey teams exposed to the same information at the same time differed in their interpretations.

Design and Methods: The protocol for simultaneous surveys consists of having one in-region and one out-of-region team survey a facility together.

Results: The regular and simultaneous survey teams generally agreed about the number of deficiencies. The intraclass correlation coefficient was 0.87 for total deficiencies and 0.76 for deficiencies with scores of G or higher. But in a substantial number of instances the teams did not agree about the scope and severity of the deficiency or about what regulation the nursing home had breached.

Implications: The survey process is reliable when assessing aggregate results, but it is only moderately reliable when examining individual citations. Stakeholders (i.e., consumers, policy makers, nursing home administrators) should be aware of the limitations of the survey process. It needs to be modified to reduce variability.

Key Words: Federal citations, F tags, Quality of care, Deficiencies

In order to participate in Medicare and Medicaid, nursing facilities must meet conditions of participation set by the Centers for Medicare and Medicaid Services (CMS; for a review, see Mullan & Harrington, 2001). In order to ensure compliance with 189 federal regulations,

[1] Address correspondence to Robert H. Lee, Department of Health Policy and Management, University of Kansas Medical Center, Mail Stop 3044, 3901 Rainbow Boulevard, Kansas City, KS 66160. E-mail: rlee2@kumc.edu Department of Health Policy and Management, University of Kansas School of Medicine, Kansas City.]

[2] University of Kansas School of Nursing, Kansas City.

[3] Schools of Allied Health and Nursing, Center for Biostatistics and Advanced Informatics, University of Kansas Medical Center, Kansas City.

state survey agencies must inspect each nursing facility every 9 to 15 months (CMS, 2005). These regulations fall into several categories: resident rights, quality of life, quality of care, resident assessment, services, dietary, pharmacy, rehabilitation, dental and physician, physical environment, and administration. Surveyors cite deficiencies when a facility does not substantially comply with a regulation. Although the regulations and survey process are federally mandated, state agencies carry out the survey process.

Dissatisfaction with the survey process is widespread. Resident advocacy groups stress that state survey teams often miss important problems with care and fail to respond to complaints quickly. A Government Accountability Office (GAO; 2004) study identified several reasons for these shortcomings: insufficient and inexperienced survey staff, confusion about the regulations, inadequate state oversight of the survey process, and the predictable timing of surveys. Surveyors question the integrity of the inspection, political pressures to water down inspection findings, and the effectiveness of the enforcement process (Grassley, 2004). Industry representatives argue that the current survey and enforcement system "is an entirely subjective, process-oriented snapshot inspection system that focuses on punishment—not quality improvement" (Ousley, 2001 p. 1).

An ongoing concern for all of these stakeholders is that the number of deficiencies varies substantially between states (GAO, 2003). For example, in 2001 the proportion of deficiency-free nursing homes ranged from 33.5% in Virginia to 0% in Nevada, and the mean number of deficiencies ranged from a high of 14.2 per facility in Nevada to a low of 1.9 per facility in New Jersey (Office of the Inspector General, 2003).

Variation also exists within states. For example, the state of Kansas is composed of 6 survey regions. In 2001 facilities in the Northeast Region averaged 11.64 deficiencies, nearly three times as many as facilities in the West Region (3.69 deficiencies). Furthermore, deficiencies in the Northeast Region tended to be assigned higher scope and severity. Administrators and directors of nursing tended to think this heterogeneity reflected differences in the survey process; surveyors thought it reflected differences in facility characteristics. Although they did not resolve this question, our earlier analyses found statistically significant regional differences ($p<.001$) even after controlling for size, case mix, nursing hours per resident day, and ownership (Forbes- Thompson et al., 2003). The reliability of the survey process appears to be worthy of careful study.

The purpose of this study was to evaluate in some depth how and why Kansas survey teams varied in their assessments. More specifically, our aim was to compare the findings of two survey teams exposed to the same information at the same point in time. We addressed this aim using a mixture of quantitative and qualitative methods.

An overview of the survey process provides a context for our study. Surveys entail standard procedures plus flexibility once a team enters a nursing facility. The process begins with presurvey preparation that includes a review of the facility's quality indicators (Arling, Kane, Lewis, & Mueller, 2005), history of complaints, and previous survey results. The team then proceeds to an entrance conference with the administrator and an initial tour. After this the team selects a group of residents, based on pre- survey information and the initial tour, for a more in- depth review. Using protocols established by CMS, the survey team gathers information in a number of ways, including medical record reviews, observations of direct resident care, resident interviews, family interviews, and observations of events such as activities and meals. Each phase of the survey process has detailed written guidelines, and as information is gathered, the team reviews it and sharpens the focus of the survey on potential problem areas.

This structure allows teams to react to and explore problems identified during data collection. It also allows for prioritization of problems while on site. However, this flexibility may also increase the variability of the survey process, because surveys of apparently similar facilities may focus on quite different aspects of care. How detailed a survey becomes also may depend on the observational skills of the surveyors, the clinical and management skills of the surveyors, or the number of problems found.

On the last day of the survey, surveyors meet to interpret their findings and to identify the number, scope, and severity of deficiencies that they found. The survey team then meets with the administrative staff and shares its preliminary findings. In Kansas, a quality improvement coordinator reviews these findings before the team submits the final survey report to the Department on Aging.

Table 1. Scope and Severity Matrix

	Scope of the Deficiency, Rating (State Share)		
Severity of the Deficiency	**Isolated**	**Pattern**	**Widespread**
Immediate jeopardy to resident health or safety	J (0.2%)	K (0.0%)	L (0.0%)
Actual harm that is not immediate jeopardy	G (5.8%)	H (0.0%)	I (0.0%)
No actual harm with potential for more than minimal harm that is not immediate jeopardy	D (45.0%)	E (34.0%)	F (9.7%)
No actual harm with potential for minimal harm	A (0.0%)	B (0.9%)	C (4.3%)

Notes: The State Share is the percentage of deficiency citations with this scope and seerity cited in surveys of freestanding Kansas nursing homes in 2003. F, H, I, J, K and L deficiencies may constitute substandard quality of care. Fines may be levied or restrictions on participation in Medicare and Medicaid may be imposed.

We should note that the final survey report may not be "final." Nursing homes can appeal any deficiencies or penalties through an informal dispute resolution process. Reductions in the number, scope, and severity of citations are common (GAO, 2003a).

Some deficiencies identify more serious problems than others, and some deficiencies allow for the imposition of more serious penalties. Table 1 outlines the scope and severity of deficiencies that surveyors may cite. Ratings A through C indicate substantial compliance with recommendations, so only Category 1 remedies are permitted (Office of the Inspector General, 2005). These remedies include development of a plan to correct the problem, enhanced monitoring by the survey agency, or mandatory training. Teams often do not cite such deficiencies. There were 0 A citations in Kansas in 2003, 21 B citations, and 96 C citations.

Citations that are rated D, E, or G permit imposition of Category Two remedies. These remedies include fines, denials of payment for new admissions, or denials of payment for all residents. These are the most common types of citations. More than 1,700 D and E deficiencies were cited in Kansas in 2003. G deficiencies are far less frequent; only 129 were issued in 2003.

Deficiencies that are rated F, H, I, J, K, or L can result in Category Three remedies. These include fines, termination from Medicare and Medicaid, and temporary management by an individual chosen by the state agency. F deficiencies are fairly common; more than 200 were cited in 2003. In contrast, H–L deficiencies are uncommon. A total of 5 J deficiencies were cited in 2003.

In most instances, the Department on Aging imposes Category Two or Three penalties only when a nursing home has failed to make corrections by the time of its resurvey. As a result, Category Two or Three penalties are not common. During the second and third quarters of 2003, the Kansas Department on Aging imposed fines on 11 nursing homes and admission bans on 18 (Kansas Department on Aging, 2004). The Department did not terminate any nursing homes from Medicaid or install temporary management in any nursing homes.

Table 2. Simultaneous Survey Protocol

Protocol
1. The RST guided all aspects of the survey process and followed normal policies and procedures.
2. RST assignments (e.g., who would conduct the closed record review) were shared with the SST so that the respective team members would be informed of their responsibilities.
3. All team meetings to discuss findings were held in separate locations and tape recorded for evaluation by the research team.
4. Preliminary off-site preparation was conducted in separate locations. The SST received the same presurvey documents to review as the RST.
5. The RST and SST were matched teams and respective SST members followed respective RST members one on one.
6. Team members were not allowed to discuss assessments or interpretations with members of the other team.
7. If the RST did not raise a concern, the SST was not allowed to pursue that issue. The SST was to document the issue in field notes.
8. Members of the SST followed respective RST members continuously (e.g., into residents' rooms to observe care and into meetings to interview staff).
9. All survey-related information (e.g., policies and procedures) were requested by and directed to the RST. Copies were made for the SST.
10. Teams and facilities were informed that the findings of the SST were not related to the facility's certification and state licensure.

Notes: RST=regular survey team; SST=simultaneous survey team.

The Department also recommended additional federal penalties to CMS.

Methods

Setting and Sample

Kansas has six geographical survey regions. Each region has at least two trained survey teams, a quality improvement coordinator, and a regional manager.

During the summer of 2003, we randomly selected two nursing homes from each region from a list of facilities scheduled for resurvey. We excluded from consideration nursing homes with fewer than 50 beds in order to reduce the burden on small facilities of having two survey teams in their home. Twelve homes comprised the sample for what we labeled "simultaneous surveys."

The simultaneous survey teams consisted of one in-region team (the regular survey team or RST) and one randomly selected out-of-region team (the simultaneous survey team or SST). The regional manager overseeing the annual survey selected the RST. The manager from another randomly selected region selected the SST. In order to ensure that survey differences were not due to their composition, we matched teams in size and expertise. For example, if the RST included their quality improvement coordinator, the SST also sent their quality improvement coordinator.

This design reflected two considerations. First, as we noted above, there were indications that the survey process varied by region. In order to examine this, the SST needed to come from a different survey region than the RST. Second, in order to ensure that the regular survey would be seen as valid by all interested parties, the RST needed to be assigned by the usual practice in that region. Otherwise a simultaneous survey might place a nursing home at a competitive advantage or disadvantage. Clearly, other designs might be preferable in other circumstances.

Procedures

Table 2 outlines the simultaneous survey protocol. The RST entered facilities following the normal protocol as prescribed by CMS. A member of the research team immediately informed the administrator that the SST would be following them as part of a quality improvement evaluation. A member of the research team also informed the administrator that the SST would not be interviewing staff, looking at or requesting additional records, or evaluating residents on their own. The SST would be shadowing the RST and reviewing its information. The RST directed the survey in accordance with policies and procedures. Members of the SST followed their RST counterparts to observe the same environmental dynamics; however, we did not allow the two team members to discuss interpretations or assessments with each other.

Survey teams usually meet several times during a survey to review what information they have collected to that point. These meetings then guide the remainder of the survey. For example, teams can use these meetings to decide which resident problems should be emphasized or which additional staff interviews are needed. The RST and SST conducted their meetings at the same time in different locations and tape recorded them. We had instructed SST members to document the problem areas and interviews they would follow up on if they were conducting a regular survey; we used the information obtained from both teams in order to evaluate consistency and provide insights into decision-making processes that influenced survey results. A member of the research team was onsite to ensure that the RST and SST members followed the protocol and did not share information with one another.

Protocol Rationale

We took several issues into consideration when designing this protocol. One was to avoid compromising the quality of resident care. Survey teams tend to disrupt normal routines, and we were concerned that repeated inspections would lead to repeated disruptions. In addition, our primary goal was to evaluate the performance of two teams exposed to the same information. Because nursing homes must address violations that teams observe during the course of an inspection, having back-to-back surveys would not have guaranteed that a follow-up survey team would have been exposed to the same problems. Conducting simultaneous surveys minimized disruption and ensured that both teams analyzed the same information.

Data Analysis

Our aim was to describe how and why the conclusions of the RST and SST differed. We used a triangulated design using both quantitative and qualitative methods (Fielding & Fielding, 1986; Jick, 1979). Our analysis of how the conclusions differed was largely quantitative. We designed the qualitative analyses to add depth to the analyses and to help answer why the reports of the teams differed.

Our approach examined the data at two very different levels of aggregation. First, treating each nursing home facility as a random effect, we calculated the intraclass correlation coefficient (ICC). The ICC equals the between-facility variance divided by the sum of the within-facility variance (from RST and SST) plus the between-facilities variance. Perfect agreement between the two survey teams would result in an ICC of 1.0, and complete randomness would result in an ICC of 0.0. Recognizing that differences in the scope and severity of deficiencies matter as well as the number of deficiencies, we cross-tabulated the deficiencies by the levels of harm cited by the RST and SST and calculated a Kappa statistic. Kappa measures how much the agreement between the teams exceeds the amount expected by chance. Complete agreement would give a Kappa of 1.0, and agreement that is no better than chance would give a Kappa of 0.0.

In order to assess why the conclusions differed, we performed a content analysis (Weber, 1990). Two registered nurse researchers, one with formal training in the survey process, independently reviewed the content of all of the written documentation for each team (researcher field notes, team notes, and meeting transcripts). They then met to resolve any differences in their reviews. In order to ensure confidentiality, we substituted numbers for resident names in these materials, and we restricted access to the materials to the research team.

In order to explore what prompted differences between the teams, the content analysis examined the data that the RST and SST used to reach their conclusions. At issue was whether the teams described different problems or characterized the same problems in different ways. For the same infraction, for example, one team could cite F-tag F221 "no unnecessary physical restraints" and another team could cite F-tag F223 "free from abuse." If both registered nurse researchers agreed that the RST and SST had cited the facility for separate shortcomings, they categorized the F tag as "distinctly different."

Table 3. Deficiencies Cited by the RST and the SST

Facility	Total Deficiencies		Gþ Deficiencies[a]		Same F Tag, Different Scope or Severity	Distinctly Different F Tags
	RST	SST	RST	SST		
1	22	23	2	2	5	14
2	3	3	0	0	1	0
3	30	31	3	5	6	14
4	9	19	0	1	4	11
5	16	24	0	1	9	11
6	17	17	2	1	7	6
7	19	15	0	1	4	5
8	18	23	1	2	6	15
9	8	9	1	1	1	7
10	13	16	0	0	6	7
11	0	1	0	0	0	1
12	6	3	0	0	0	5
Total	161	187	9	14	49	96
Intraclass correlation coefficient		0.87		0.76		
95% confidence interval	0.64–0.96		0.38–0.92			

Notes: RST = regular survey team; SST = simultaneous survey team.
[a] G+ deficiencies include G, H, I, J, K, and L, but none higher than H were cited.

Results

ICCs

Table 3 shows that the RST and SST cited similar numbers of deficiencies. The ICC for total deficiencies cited by the two teams was 0.87 with a 95% confidence interval of 0.64 to 0.96. Given that values greater than 0.70 indicate good reliability, this is quite high (Kramer & Feinstein, 1981). The RST and SST also cited similar numbers of G+ deficiencies. The ICC was 0.76 with a 95% confidence interval of 0.38 to 0.92. The SST cited more deficiencies than the RST for 8 of the 12 nursing homes, but a paired t test failed to reject the hypothesis that the means were the same.

Counts do not fully describe the decisions of the RST and SST. Table 3 also shows that in 49 instances the RST and SST agreed about which regulation was being breached but differed on the scope and severity. In another 96 instances, the two teams cited distinctly different deficiencies, meaning that they identified different failures to comply with the regulations. The number of distinctly different deficiencies rose with the number of citations. The correlation with RST citations was 0.76 and the correlation with SST citations was 0.89. Both correlations were significantly different from 0 at the 0.01 level.

Kappa Statistics

Table 4 cross-tabulates the findings of the RST and SST, focusing on the levels of harm identified. With 12 facilities and 189 regulations, 2,268 violations were possible. Overall, the level of agreement was moderate, as we estimated a Kappa of 0.57 (Landis & Koch, 1977). Kappa estimates the degree of consensus while controlling for the amount of chance agreement to be expected based on the marginal distributions (Stemler, 2004). Because the RST and SST found no deficiencies most of the time, we needed this control in order to avoid overstating reliability.

In most instances neither team found a violation. The RST found no violations 92.9% of the time, and the SST found no violations 91.8% of the time. The SST agreed with the RST 96.5% of the time.

The teams seldom cited deficiencies entailing no actual harm with potential for minimal harm. The RST gave 11 A, B, or C citations, and the SST gave 9. The similar totals masked considerable disagreement. The SST found no deficiency for 55% of the A–C deficiencies cited by the RST and found a D–F deficiency for 18%. The RST found no deficiency for 11% of the A–C deficiencies cited by the SST and found a D–F deficiency for 56%.

Table 4. Cross-Tabulations of Deficiencies by Level of Harm

Deficiency	No Deficiency	A–C	D–F	G–I	J–L	RST Totals
No deficiency	2,033	1	69	4	0	2,107
A–C	6	3	2	0	0	11
D–F	41	5	89	6	0	141
G–I	1	0	4	4	0	9
J–L	0	0	0	0	0	0
SST totals	2,081	9	164	14	0	2,268

Notes: RST = regular survey team; SST = simultaneous survey team.

A–C deficiencies find no actual harm with potential for minimal harm. D–F deficiencies find no actual harm with po¬tential for more than minimal harm. G–I deficiencies find actual harm for residents. J–L deficiencies find immediate jeopardy for residents.

Kappa = 0.57.

Deficiencies with D–F scope and severity levels, which entail a finding of no actual harm with the potential for more than minimal harm, were the most common citations. Most disagreements also involved these deficiencies. Of the 141 cited by the RST, the SST cited no deficiency for 29%, an A–C deficiency for 4%, a D–F for 63%, and a G–I for 4%. Of the 164 D–F deficiencies cited by the SST, the RST cited no deficiency for 42%, an A–C deficiency for 1%, a D–F deficiency for 54%, and a G–I for 2%. In short, both teams cited no deficiency in a substantial number of the cases in which the other team issued a D–F deficiency.

Deficiencies involving actual harm were uncommon. Even so, the teams differed in their conclusions. The SST cited a D–F deficiency for 4 of the 9 G–I deficiencies cited by the RST and found no breach of the remaining regulation. The RST cited a D–F deficiency for 6 of the 14 G–I deficiencies cited by the SST and found no breach in four instances.

Neither team cited J, K, or L deficiencies, which involve immediate jeopardy for residents.

Content Analysis

As noted above, ICC and Kappa calculations do not fully take into account the differences between the RST and SST. A closer examination of Facility 6 illustrates this. The RST and SST cited the same number of deficiencies, yet there were important differences in their findings. In seven instances the teams disagreed on the scope and severity of the deficiencies, and in six instances the teams cited distinctly different deficiencies. Most of the scope and severity differences were minor, but not all. The RST and SST both identified quality of care deficiencies in the management of pain. The RST assigned an E deficiency, and the SST assigned a G, implying actual harm to residents. The RST and SST both identified deficiencies in the treatment of residents with pressure ulcers. The RST assigned a G deficiency, and the SST assigned a D. In addition, the RST cited three deficiencies that the SST did not: not having an adequate activities program, improperly ordering medications, and not having a backup power supply system. The SST cited four deficiencies that the RST did not: failing to reassess a resident whose condition had changed, not taking adequate care to prevent urinary tract infections, having an overly high medication error rate, and failing to investigate a bruise of unknown origin.

Some disagreements reflected different interpretations of the facts, even though the RST shaped the information that both teams had. For example, in Facility 4 the RST issued a D quality of care citation because the facility failed to follow its own protocol in caring for a resident with a pressure ulcer. The SST identified additional problems with the care provided to this resident and saw similar problems in the care of another resident. The SST issued a G quality of care citation. In another instance, both the RST and SST cited Facility 3 for failures to provide an appropriate accounting of resident funds. The initial citations were both Es, but the SST ultimately assigned an H. The difference appeared to spring from the conclusion of the SST that at least three items that had been purchased with residents' funds could not be found anywhere in the facility, an issue that the RST did not address. The SST issued an additional H citation for staff treatment of residents and revised its citation for improper accounting of resident funds citation to an H.

Overall, SSTs cited 26 more deficiencies than RSTs, with 18 of these coming from Facilities 4 and 5. For Facility 4, the SST final report identified 10 more deficiencies than the RST final report. The SST issued seven D citations for problems that the RST did not identify or discuss. The SST also issued two citations for problems that the RST combined into one deficiency. After consultation with the regional office, the RST chose not to cite two problems that both teams had identified. In one instance the RST discussed a problem that the SST cited, but decided not to cite the facility. (The RST also cited one deficiency that the SST did not.) For Facility, 5 the SST identified eight more deficiencies than the RST. Five of these deficiencies were due to inconsistencies between the care plan and the care provided that the SST examined and the RST did not. The missing care included activities for one resident, assistance with eating for another resident, protective booties for a resident at risk for pressure ulcers, a contracture boot for another resident, and range of motion therapy for yet another resident.

Our observers noted a striking difference in how the teams tracked medication administration. In Facility 4 the RST focused on one of the medications given to a resident, but the SST made notes on all of the resident's medications. The two teams found similar numbers of errors, but the SST calculated a much lower error rate because the denominator was much larger. The RST gave an E deficiency to Facility 4 for medication administration; the SST did not.

In their discussions, SST members critiqued the RST fairly regularly. For example, the SST notes for Facility 6 included comments that, "I would have followed up more on [the] broken thermostat," and "I would have knocked and checked" to see if a resident scheduled for an interview was in her room with the door closed. The SST notes for Facility 11 noted that there were unasked questions about a "resident being left alone on toilet and orthostatic hypotension" and "fall investigation." Additionally, some teams identified deficiencies by "running through the regulations." Other teams identified deficiencies by running through the leader's concerns.

Yet attributing these differences to the teams obscures the important roles of other staff.

Teams discuss concerns with their regional managers and quality improvement coordinators several times during a survey. Furthermore, teams discuss their findings with these administrative staff following their decision-making meeting. Again, this process has both strengths and weaknesses. On the one hand, the experience of regional managers and quality improvement coordinators allows them to assist more junior surveyors by providing guidance and putting information into perspective. On the other hand, most regional managers and quality improvement coordinators are not on site and so provide guidance without seeing the evidence firsthand. Analyses of meeting and field notes indicated that the number of changes between the initial and final reports ranged from 0 to 14 per team.

Several comments indicated that regional managers had a significant influence on the survey process. For example, some regional managers did not encourage surveyors to write deficiencies for paperwork violations unless there were concomitant care problems. In addition, some surveyors noted that their regional managers instructed them that hand washing had to be a huge issue before they should cite it. One team commented that their regional manager would never let them go into an extended survey for a particular F tag. Some teams made a point of staying for the first meal after entering the facility, and others did not. Some teams were very methodical in their decision-making style, going in order through the regulations, whereas others discussed concerns according to their priority or in top-of-mind order. In short, different teams used different processes.

An important finding was that teams differed in assessments of scope and severity for the same resident care issue. Our content analysis identified several instances in which there were no clear right or wrong assessments of scope and severity. When teams disagreed on the scope and severity, we could trace these differences to differences in interpretations of the regulations and of the interventions provided by the facility.

An example dealing with pressure ulcer prevention and healing illustrates the difficulty with scope and severity determinations. The *Facility Guide to OBRA Regulations, and Interpretive Guidelines and the LTC Survey Process* offers the following guidance:

> A determination that development of a pressure sore was unavoidable may be made only if routine preventive and daily care was provided. Routine preventive care means turning and proper positioning, application of pressure reduction or relief devices, providing good skin care, (i.e., keeping the skin clean, instituting measures to reduce excessive moisture), providing clean and dry bed linens, and maintaining adequate nutrition and hydration as possible. (p. 22)

Their notes indicated that surveyors seldom had difficulty in determining whether the facility identified the resident as being at risk. But surveyors looking at the same evidence disagreed on whether the facility interventions were aggressive enough or whether the facility tried enough different interventions. Surveyors scrutinized the data collected and took their decisions very seriously but had differing perceptions of when a facility had done enough.

Discussion

Even though the teams examined the same data, they often differed in the number, scope, and severity of deficiencies cited. The teams also routinely assigned different F tags when they cited facilities. In short, the teams generated substantially different surveys from the same facts. Yet abstracting from the details of the surveys, the teams painted very similar pictures of facilities' overall compliance with federal regulations.

These data support two very different interpretations. One stresses the variability of the survey process; the other stresses its global consistency. The variability interpretation notes that the two survey teams often reached different conclusions about whether a deficiency existed, what regulation had been breached, the scope of the deficiency, or the severity of the deficiency. These differences, furthermore, might well have consequences. The penalties imposed by the survey agency, the career prospects of facility managers, and the responses of consumers are likely to be different for a nursing home that gets 7 D deficiencies than for a nursing home that gets 12 D deficiencies and 1 G.

The variability of the survey process reduces its value to nursing home managers, who should be the primary users of its detailed findings. The same process can draw no deficiencies from one survey team and multiple deficiencies from another. As a result, nursing home administrators and directors of nursing cannot be confident that a good survey means that a process works well. Nor can administrators and directors of nursing be confident that genuine improvements in care will result in a better survey if the next team relies on different interpretations of the regulations and what constitutes having done enough. Speaking for a number of her peers, one director of nursing described the survey process as "demoralizing." Improvement efforts are inhibited by a survey process that falls short of systematic, replicable data gathering and analysis (Schnelle, Osterweil, & Simmons, 2005).

The variability of the survey also reduces its value to regulators and policy makers. The inspection is supposed to provide assurance that a nursing home is in substantial compliance with federal and state regulations, either at the time of the inspection or after completion of a plan to correct problems. An unreliable survey process may mean that nursing homes that do not actually meet federal or state standards will be eligible for Medicare and Medicaid payments. The many disagreements of these two teams about whether a regulation had been breached, which regulation had been breached, and how serious the breach was cannot make federal or state officials comfortable.

The variability perspective would also note that we had designed the structure of this study in order to exclude some forms of variation. Had they not been constrained to look at the data assembled by the RST, the members of the SST might well have gathered different facts and identified different problems. Indeed, comments to this effect by members of the SST were routine. It is likely that this study understates the variability of the survey process.

Yet these data also highlight the overall consistency of the survey results. The total numbers of deficiencies and the number of G+ deficiencies cited by the RST and SST were quite similar. If consumers rely on the total number of deficiencies or the number of high-level deficiencies as measures of quality, our results suggest that consumers should view surveys as highly reliable. We do not know how consumers use nursing home survey results, but their structure suggests that consumers should use them as part of a broader assessment process. Surveys may not reflect current conditions in a nursing home and should be used with care, just like any other measure.

Viewed at a macro level, this study suggests that, given the same data, the two teams reached very similar conclusions. Viewed at a micro level, this study suggests just the opposite. Although state survey agencies and consumers may feel comfortable focusing on macro results, managers must make decisions at the micro level, and their concerns about reliability weaken the credibility of the survey process. In order to reduce the variability of survey results, changes in the survey process and in the training of surveyors warrant consideration. The CMS trial of the Quality Indicator Survey appears to be a promising initiative (CMS, 2004). This five-state experiment enhances training, sampling, and decision support software to make surveys more structured.

This article suggests that surveyors need more specific criteria, in the form of decision-making algorithms, to reduce the influence of individual perceptions. These findings concur with other evaluations of survey consistency (GAO, 2003b; Office of the Inspector General, 2003, 2004). CMS has begun a process of developing and evaluating clearer guidelines for surveyors. Our findings support that effort.

These results also suggest that continued efforts to standardize training and decision rules are important. Especially at the state level, common understandings of what constitutes a breach of the regulations should reduce the angst of the industry and increase the confidence of regulators and the public. In assigning the number, scope, and severity of deficiencies, consistency is of primary importance.

One should not overlook the limitations of this study. It applies to one state with a specific administrative structure. Moreover, the sample used in this study was not large. And, although they were randomly selected and generated data comparable to statewide averages, we cannot guarantee that the facilities or survey teams were representative of Kansas. The results should not be generalized to other states. Furthermore, this study eliminated differences in the information collected. As a result, the differences reported here were entirely due to differences in interpretation. As we noted above, these results seem likely to understate the variability of survey results in the wild.

It is important to remember that the survey process is designed to measure compliance with federal regulations. It is tempting to infer that a survey with few deficiencies identifies a good facility and a survey with many deficiencies identifies a bad one. Indeed, numerous research studies and consumer guides do exactly that (e.g., Castle, 2000; Castle & Mor, 1998; Harrington, O'Meara, Kitchener, Simon, & Schnelle, 2003). Yet, as one surveyor noted, "The number of deficiencies is not a good quality indicator for whether I would put my mom somewhere or not. You know it relates back to what was the scope and severity of those deficiencies and what were those deficiencies really about" Our results suggest that the survey process is only moderately reliable in describing the scope and severity of nursing home deficiencies. Given that compliance with federal regulations may well have changed since the survey was completed, consumers should use the survey results with care.

Many states and CMS rely on public reporting of survey results as a spur to better nursing home care. Indeed, this appears to represent an important de facto shift from a policy of pure deterrence to a policy of deterrence plus transparency (Chou, 2002). Consumers evidently seek this information. Yahoo! reports that "Nursing Home Compare" is the nation's second most popular nursing home care site and is one of the most frequently visited sections of the Medicare Web site (Office of the Inspector General, 2004; Yahoo! Health Directory, 2005). As a result, the reliability of nursing home surveys becomes an even more visible public policy issue. Survey results will have the greatest impact on nursing home quality if consumers and the industry believe that deficiencies are valid, reliable measures of quality. This belief will be undercut by variations in the number, scope, and severity of deficiencies when the facts are held constant. The appropriate policy response is to acknowledge these variations and address them by clarifying definitions and interpretations, by improving training, and by providing feedback to surveyors. Simultaneous surveys like the ones reported here should become standard features of survey agencies. Using simultaneous surveys as a calibration tool is clearly feasible.

REFERENCES

Arling, G., Kane, R. L., Lewis, T., & Mueller, C. (2005). Future development of nursing home quality indicators. *The Gerontologist*, *45*, 147–156.

Castle, N. (2000). Nursing homes increasing and decreasing restraint use. *Medical Care*, *38*, 1154–1163.

Castle, N., & Mor, V. (1998). The use of physical restraints in nursing homes: A review of the literature since the Nursing Home Reform Act. *Medical Care Research and Review*, *55*, 139–170.

Centers for Medicare and Medicaid Services. (2004). *Action plan for nursing home quality. Retrieved August 25, 2005*, from http://www.cms.hhs.gov/ quality/nhqi/ NHActionPlan.pdf

Centers for Medicare and Medicaid Services. (2005). *The official U.S. government site for people with Medicare*. Retrieved June 15, 2005, from http://www.medicare.gov

Chou, S. (2002). Asymmetric information, ownership and quality of care: An empirical analysis of nursing homes. *Journal of Health Economics*, *21*, 293–311.

Fielding, N. G., & Fielding, J. L. (1986). *Linking data: The articulation of qualitative and quantitative methods in social research*. Beverly Hills: Sage.

Forbes-Thompson, S., Dunton, N., Gajewski, B., Wrona, M., Becker, A., Chapin, R., et al. (2003). *Kansas nursing facility project evaluation*. Kansas City: Kansas Department of Aging.

Government Accountability Office. (2003a). *Nursing home deficiency trends and survey and certification process consistency*. Retrieved October 11, 2006, from http://oig.hhs.gov/oei/reports/oei-02-01-00600.pdf

Government Accountability Office. (2003b). *Nursing home quality: Prevalence of serious problems, while declining, reinforces importance of enhanced oversight* (Report No. GAO-03-561). Retrieved June 15, 2005, from http://www.gao.gov/ new.items/d031016t.pdf

Government Accountability Office. (2004). *Prevalence of serious quality problems remains unacceptably high, despite some decline* (Report No. GAO-03-1016T). Retrieved June 15, 2005, from http://www.gao. gov/new.items/d031 01 6t.pdf

Grassley, C. R. & Letter to Mark McClellan. (July 7, 2004). Retrieved October 11, 2006 from http://www.canhr.org/news/GrassleyLetter. html#LetterToCMS.

Harrington, C., O'Meara, J., Kitchener, M., Simon, L. P., & Schnelle, J. F. (2003). Designing a report card for nursing facilities: What information is needed and why. *The Gerontologist, 43*(Special Issue II), 47–57.

Jick, T. D. (1979). Mixing qualitative and quantitative methods: Triangulation in action. *Administrative Science Quarterly, 24*, 602–611.

Kansas Department on Aging. (2004). Sunflower connection. Retrieved May 8, 2006, from http://www.agingkansas.org/kdoa/lce/facts_newsltr/ jan_2004_final.pdf

Kramer, M., & Feinstein, A. (1981). The biostatistics of concordance. *Clinical Pharmacology and Therapeutics, 29*, 111–123.

Landis, J., & Koch, G. (1977). The measurement of observer agreement for categorical data. *Biometrics, 33*, 159–174.

Mullan, J. T., & Harrington, C. (2001). Nursing home deficiencies in the United States. *Research on Aging, 23*, 503–531.

Office of the Inspector General. (2003). *Nursing home deficiency trends and survey and certification process consistency*. Retrieved February 24, 2006, from http://oig.hhs.gov/oei/reports/oei-02-01-00600.pdf

Office of the Inspector General. (2004). *Inspection results on Nursing Home Compare: Completeness and accuracy*. Retrieved August 18, 2005, from http://www.canhr.org/ pdfs/oei-01-03-00130.pdf

Office of the Inspector General. (2005). *Nursing home enforcement: The use of civil monetary penalties*. Retrieved February 24, 2006, from http://oig.hhs.gov/oei/reports/oei-06-02-00720.pdf

Ousley, M. K. (2001). *Testimony before the Subcommittee on Health of the House Committee on Ways and Means*, March 15, 2001. Retrieved June 15, 2005, from http://waysandmeans.house.gov/legacy/health/ 1 07cong/3-15-01 /3-15ous.htm

Pate, T. (2005). T*he Facility Guide to OBRA Regulations and the Long- Term Care Survey Process*. Miamisburg, OH: Med-Pass.

Schnelle, J. F., Osterweil, D., & Simmons, S. F. (2005). Improving the quality of nursing home care and medical-record accuracy with direct observational technologies. *The Gerontologist, 45*, 576–582.

Stemler, S. E. (2004). A comparison of consensus, consistency, and measurement approaches to estimating interrater reliability. *Practical Assessment, Research & Evaluation, 9*(4). Retrieved March 9, 2006, from http://PAREonline.net/getvn.asp?v=9&n=4

Weber, R. P. (1990). *Basic content analysis* (2nd ed.). Newbury Park, CA: Sage.

Yahoo! Health Directory. (2005). *Site listings by popularity*. Retrieved August 17, 2005, from http://dir.yahoo.com/Health/Long_Term_Care/ Nursing_Home_Care/

End Notes

[1] See, e.g., Lee, Gajewski & Thompson, "Reliability of the Nursing Home Survey Process: A Simultaneous Survey Approach," 46 THE GERONTOLOGIST 772-780 (2006) (copy attached to testimony).

[2] There is extensive literature on quality but it is not easily accessible to consumers. "Aging Services: The Not-For-Profit Difference", an AAHSA publication, cites many of these independent studies as identifying higher quality provided by NFPs.

[3] Other organizations that have developed consumer guides include the American Health Care Association (AHCA) and NCCNHR, the nursing home consumer advocacy organization.

[4] Quality First is the industry-wide voluntary quality improvement initiative initiated in 2001 by AAHSA, AHCA and the Alliance (which represents publicly-traded nursing home companies). The associations implement Quality First independently.

[5] Not-for-profits are obligated to report their finances to the IRS on the I-990 form, make the form publicly available, and meet specific governance and charitable requirements to maintain their tax exempt status. It should be noted that publicly traded companies are also required to report their finances and major business activities; it is the financial obligations that are significantly different.

[6] Lee, et al., "If at First You Don't Succeed: Efforts to Improve Collaboration Between Nursing Homes and a Health System", Topics in Advanced Nursing eJournal, www.medscape.com (posted 09/01/94).

[7] Hunt, *A Family Caregiver's Guide to Hospital Discharge Planning* is available at www.strengthforcaring.com.

[8] Marquardt Memorial adapted many of the elements of the various culture transformation models to meet our community's needs. It is not necessary to adopt an entire program; what is necessary is the will to create a healthy nursing home workplace and to maintain that healthy workplace over the years.

[9] The "Patient Safety" movement, building on the seminal Institute of Medicine studies of hospital errors, provides a good starting point for shifting from a "blame" mode to a "fix the problem" mode – in many respects the culture change movement in nursing homes, described above, addresses the recommendations made by IOM and safety experts. AAHSA staff would be happy to discuss this in greater depth with the Committee.

In: Nursing Homes Quality and Care Issues
Editor: Carlos E. Melendez
ISBN: 978-1-61668-855-4

Chapter 11

NURSING HOME TRANSPARENCY, ENFORCEMENT & QUALITY IMPROVEMENT HEARING*

David R. Zimmerman

Good Afternoon.

My name is David Zimmerman. I am a Professor of Health Systems Engineering in the Department of Industrial and Systems Engineering at the University of Wisconsin-Madison, and I am the Director of the Center for Health Systems Research and Analysis at UW-Madison. I am also the President of the Long Term Care Institute, a non-profit organization created to assist in the monitoring of quality of nursing home care in organizations with Corporate Integrity Agreements with the DHHS Office of the Inspector General.

I have been conducting research in nursing home quality of care and performance measurement for 25 years. Researchers at our center have been involved in CMS-funded efforts to improve the quality assurance process for more than a decade. We also developed the original set of quality indicators based on the Minimum Data Set, as well as the software to make the data on these indicators available to all 17,000 nursing homes and all 50 state survey agencies. More recently, as part of our work on corporate integrity agreements with the DHHS OIG, we at the Long Term Care Institute have been involved in 13 monitoring engagements with national and regional corporations under OIG corporate integrity agreements, covering more than 1000 nursing homes and 100,000 nursing home residents.

In the combination of these activities, our clinicians and systems analysts have conducted visits to more than 900 nursing homes in the past six years. We have observed or participated in more than 100 quality improvement meetings, including more than 30 such sessions at the corporate level of organizations. I have spoken to at least 15 corporate boards or board committees and met with individual board members about quality of care issues.

---

* This is an edited, reformatted and augmented version of a U. S. Senate Special Committee on Aging publication dated November 15, 2007.

These activities have given us important insights into the world of quality assurance and quality improvement in nursing homes and the corporations that own some of them. They also provide the basis for some observations and suggestions for ways that the federal government can truly protect the health and safety of nursing home residents, perhaps the most vulnerable population in our society. Below I have set forth some suggested legislative solutions to improve nursing home quality of care.

There has been increasing attention focused on the quality of nursing home care, most recently because of the rise in the number of ownership transactions between regional and large nursing home corporations, and the tendency for these transactions to involve a transfer of ownership from a public corporation to entities commonly referred to as private equity firms. At the heart of this debate and scrutiny is a corollary issue that should, in fact, be the center of our attention, and that I fear is being lost in the scuffles over private equity ownership. That issue is **transparency**.

Solution 1: There should be complete transparency on full ownership of every nursing home.

It should be undeniable that the purchaser and recipient of nursing home care have the right to know who is providing that care. When that purchaser is the federal government, which spends billions of dollars on nursing home care every year, the case for complete transparency is compelling. Simply put, the federal government should have the right to know, with complete transparency, the complete ownership structure of every nursing home participating in the Medicare and Medicaid program. This should be true no matter which or what type of entity owns them. There are several corollary principles that follow from the right to ownership transparency:

1. The complete ownership structure of all entities involved in the provision and administration of resident care should be fully reported to CMS.
2. The ownership reporting requirement should be the responsibility of the provider organization. The provider organization should set forth, in understandable detail, the complete ownership of all parties involved in the provision and administration of resident care.
3. The principle of transparency should apply no matter what level of complexity in the labyrinth of organizational structures exists. In fact, the more complex the web, the greater the need for more detailed transparency. And, the greater the complexity, the more reasonable it is that the originator of that complexity ought to have the responsibility for explaining it to the purchaser of care.

Solution 2: Staffing information for every nursing home should be reported in a standardized format.

In addition to ownership transparency, there should be transparency on the staffing in nursing homes. In the world of health systems, we often describe the nature of the work along two dimensions: "tech"(nology) and "touch." In an industry as "high-touch" as nursing home care, it is reasonable for the purchaser of care to know the labor resources that are being devoted to that task. Nursing homes should report the staff resources, on a resident-time basis, that are devoted to resident care. This information should be based on payroll data, which exist in accessible form for virtually every nursing home in the country. The technological means exist to submit and receive staffing data, in a standardized format, for the entire nursing home industry. Reasonable people representing all stakeholders can make sound decisions about how to structure the definitions into a common taxonomy. Acuity-based staffing in this industry is far more crowed about than practiced, but these adjustments can be taken into account if necessary.

Solution 3: There needs to be greater ability to expand the scope of observation and analysis from individual facilities to nursing home corporations and networks.

Currently, virtually all regulatory activity is focused on the individual nursing home. To a large extent this is because of the concept that the "licensee" is the operator of record and accountability. Yet in many survey situations, it is the corporate entity that will be integrally involved in the process from the provider side. Related and equally important, it is often the corporation's policies and procedures that govern the system of care in the facility. In some cases these corporate policies and procedures are inadequate to provide proper governance to the delivery of care. Yet in many other cases, the problem at the facility and resident levels is that reasonable policies and procedures are not being executed consistently across facilities in the network. A stronger focus on this level of management would be a much more efficient way to improve care systematically across an organization, as opposed to one facility at a time.

Yet, currently there is virtually no way that a state regulatory agency can expand its scope across state lines. CMS does have greater authority to expand the scope to a more systematic examination of multi-facility networks, even across state lines, but much more could be done to utilize the available information in an aggregated fashion to focus on regional and even national nursing home networks. Our Center produces monthly reports on survey deficiencies comparing the largest national corporations and provides them to the OIG and to each specific corporation that is covered by a Corporate Integrity Agreement. (I have provided de-identified examples of these types of reports with this testimony.) And we provide similar information on the MDS quality indicator/quality measures to the same parties, on a quarterly basis. This information can and should be provided on all national and regional corporations on a routine basis.

In addition to the information vehicle described above, CMS should have the authority to take corrective action with respect to corporate entities if there are problems at individual facilities. More often than not, the problems found at a network's facilities display a common set of patterns and issues; it is much more efficient to deal with these issues and corrective responses on a broader basis than just individual facility actions.

Solution 4: There should be more use of intermediate corrective measures.

There have long been calls for broader and more innovative ways to incentivize, exhort, and pressure providers into taking better and more systematic corrective actions to improve care and sustain that higher care level. These appeals have continued unabated, and have actually become more urgent in recent years, because of the confluence of three very troubling trends: the demographic graying of America, the increasing complexity of the nursing home population as it accepts more post-acute patients, and the stagnant or decreasing skill sets of provider staff. Care problems need to be identified earlier and addressed—in meaningful ways—more promptly and with more ingenuity and commitment. The current arsenal of intermediate sanction weapons— including admissions freezes, civil monetary penalties, and suspension of CNA training programs—have been used to varying degree and imposed inconsistently. There needs to be more stable use of these vehicles for correction and improvement. But there also needs to be increased scrutiny on providers—at both the facility and network levels—who have not demonstrated the ability to adequately self-identify a problem and fix it; and then keep it fixed.

One measure that has demonstrated success in both process and outcomes is the use of monitors to provide additional scrutiny on the care provided in problematic facilities, as well as the systems put in place to correct identified problems and sustain the fix. Our previously mentioned work with several national corporations has provided a number of insights into the barriers to and facilitators of quality improvement efforts. In particular, the focus of attention on the corporate district level—the level of the corporation just above the individual facility level— has proven extremely valuable, improving the consistency of the quality assurance protocols and activities as they are rolled out from this level to facilities. Similarly, our focus on the ***systems*** of care delivery and quality assurance has shown both model practices and complete breakdowns in how care is provided, and how quality improvement efforts have been effective or not. Providers sometimes focus inordinate attention on finding "leaders," then expecting them to work miracles without giving them the support they need to be successful, and then holding them solely responsible if this impossible task is not accomplished. I call this the "awesome goat" phenomenon, and we have seen it in action scores of times. Monitoring can correctly place the focus on the systems of care that need to be implemented consistently across every facility, every shift, and at every bedside.

The monitoring process can promote and expand the concept of transparency described earlier. Facilities and organizations that have demonstrated problems in providing and assuring quality care will be the focus of additional attention and scrutiny, with the transparency that monitors can provide to determine the capability of the provider to improve their systems and oversight.

Solution 5: Increase the focus on the landlord as well as the licensed operator.

Currently, the entity owning the actual physical asset of the nursing home (the "bricks and mortar" as it is called) has virtually no responsibility or accountability for the adequacy of the care provided at the facility. Yet we have seen cases in which the actions (or inactions) of the landlord have had deleterious, and sometimes direct, effects on the quality of care in the facility. For example, there are sometimes restrictive clauses in the lease agreements that effectively prohibit the licensed operator from making needed upgrades or renovations consistent with evidence-based care practices. Other restrictive lease practices might make the implementation of physical or structural changes so onerous financially that it becomes prohibitive for the licensed operator to even consider such changes. It is certainly conceivable that a licensed operator might find itself in the "Catch 22" situation of being in violation of federal certification or state licensure regulations that cannot be fixed without taking steps that are legally or financially prohibitive in the lease it has with a landlord.

I realize that this problem, in particular, might be very difficult to solve. Holding the landlord to the same certification and licensing requirements of the operator may not be feasible. But consideration should be given to (a) making sure that the lease provisions are transparent, along with other aspects of ownership, and (b) finding a way to ensure that if lease agreements stand in the way of corrective actions necessary to bring about compliance with conditions of participation, there is a way to deal with these situations.

CONCLUSION

All the solutions I propose above have to do, in some way, with increasing the transparency of information about who provides care, and who owns whatever entity or entities responsible for the decisions pertaining to that care. Transparency is essential to the continued delivery of nursing home care through existing private and public markets. There is an elegant simplicity to transparency solutions. With full transparency of ownership, so we know who is and should be accountable, and transparency on staffing so we know who is providing care, we can examine the outcomes as they are produced through the survey process and examination of resident-level outcomes. Facilities and organizations demonstrating their ability to deliver adequate (and hopefully excellent) care can continue on with this critical task, and with our appreciation. Facilities and organizations that have demonstrated an inability to deliver adequate care can expect to see additional scrutiny and even greater transparency requirements, including outside monitors to assure that they can earn our trust to provide care and protect the health and safety of our most vulnerable population.

INDEX

U

V

W

X